METHODS IN MOLECULAR BIOLOGY

For further volumes:
http://www.springer.com/series/7651

Fragile-X Syndrome

Methods and Protocols

Edited by

Dalit Ben-Yosef and Yoav Mayshar

Wolfe PGD Stem Cell Lab, Racine IVF Unit at Lis Maternity Hospital, Tel Aviv Sourasky Medical Center, Tel Aviv University, Tel Aviv, Israel

Humana Press

Editors
Dalit Ben-Yosef
Wolfe PGD Stem Cell Lab, Racine IVF
Unit at Lis Maternity Hospital
Tel Aviv Sourasky Medical Center
Tel Aviv University
Tel Aviv, Israel

Yoav Mayshar
Wolfe PGD Stem Cell Lab, Racine IVF
Unit at Lis Maternity Hospital
Tel Aviv Sourasky Medical Center
Tel Aviv University
Tel Aviv, Israel

ISSN 1064-3745 ISSN 1940-6029 (electronic)
Methods in Molecular Biology
ISBN 978-1-4939-9079-5 ISBN 978-1-4939-9080-1 (eBook)
https://doi.org/10.1007/978-1-4939-9080-1

Library of Congress Control Number: 2019932993

This Humana Press imprint is published by the registered company Springer Science+Business Media, LLC, part of Springer Nature.
The registered company address is: 233 Spring Street, New York, NY 10013, U.S.A.

Preface

Fragile X syndrome (FXS) is the most common form of inherited cognitive impairment and the most common hereditary cause of autism. The syndrome is caused by inactivation of the FMR1 gene and its encoded protein FMRP, which results in defects in brain development and function. The loss of function of FMR1 is due to a CGG trinucleotide repeat expansion mutation in the 5'-UTR of the gene that is epigenetically regulated on the DNA and histone levels. Individuals with >200 CGG repeats are considered affected, and all the males among them will be affected since it is an X-linked condition. In contrast, most of the females display a milder form of the disease, and few present with the severe phenotype. For many years, the research into the molecular and cellular basis of FXS was focused mainly on knockout animals. More of the recent studies have been conducted on pluripotent stem cells (iPs and hESC) carrying the natural mutation. Neurodevelopmental disorders, such as FXS, often involve multiple cell types and molecular pathways. FXS is still poorly understood since the affected neural cell types have not yet been clearly defined, nor has the neurodevelopmental trajectory leading to the pathology been elucidated. Various in vitro neural differentiation technologies to generate different types of neural cells were developed in an effort to advance the knowledge in these areas. Neural precursor cells that are isolated from the brains of fetuses and adults are also being studied for their contribution to the development of FXS. Several chapters in this book describe these new technologies in detail.

Interestingly, individuals that carry between 55 and 200 CGG repeats and are considered as being permutation carriers are also affected with either fragile X primary ovarian insufficiency or fragile X-associated tremor/ataxia syndrome. Two chapters in this book are dedicated to the new technologies that are currently being used for exploring the pathophysiology of these conditions.

This book contains 15 chapters on the state-of-the-art technologies for investigating all aspects of FXS. It is our hope that it will motivate more scientists to study FXS and achieve the elusive goal of developing therapeutic solutions for ameliorating its symptoms and even reach the ultimate goal of discovering the long-awaited cure.

Tel Aviv, Israel

Dalit Ben-Yosef
Yoav Mayshar

Contents

Contributors

MOHAMMAD ARIF • *Department of Genetics and Genomic Sciences, Icahn School of Medicine at Mount Sinai, New York, NY, USA*
DALIT BEN-YOSEF • *Wolfe PGD Stem Cell Lab, Racine IVF Unit at Lis Maternity Hospital, Tel Aviv Sourasky Medical Center, Tel Aviv University, Tel Aviv, Israel*
ANITA BHATTACHARYYA • *Waisman Center, University of Wisconsin-Madison, Madison, WI, USA; Department of Cell and Regenerative Biology, University of Wisconsin-Madison, Madison, WI, USA*
VOLKER BUSSKAMP • *Center for Regenerative Therapies, Technische Universität Dresden, Dresden, Germany*
XIAOQIANG CAI • *Department of Genetics and Genomic Sciences, Icahn School of Medicine at Mount Sinai, New York, NY, USA; Sema4, a Mount Sinai Venture, Stamford, CT, USA; WuXi AppTec Group, Shanghai, China*
MAIJA L. CASTRÉN • *Faculty of Medicine, Physiology, University of Helsinki, Helsinki, Finland*
YORAM COHEN • *IVF unit, Department of Obstetrics and Gynecology, Chaim Sheba Medical Center (Tel Hashomer), Ramat Gan, Israel; The Fertility Research Laboratory, Chaim Sheba Medical Center (Tel Hashomer), Ramat Gan, Israel*
OLGA DRATVIMAN-STOROBINSKY • *IVF unit, Department of Obstetrics and Gynecology, Chaim Sheba Medical Center (Tel Hashomer), Ramat Gan, Israel*
LISA J. EDELMANN • *Department of Genetics and Genomic Sciences, Icahn School of Medicine at Mount Sinai, New York, NY, USA; Sema4, a Mount Sinai Venture, Stamford, CT, USA*
RACHEL EIGES • *Stem Cell Research Laboratory, Medical Genetics Institute, Shaare Zedek Medical Center, Jerusalem, Israel; Hebrew University Medical School, Jerusalem, Israel*
SHAI E. ELIZUR • *IVF unit, Department of Obstetrics and Gynecology, Chaim Sheba Medical Center (Tel Hashomer), Ramat Gan, Israel; The Fertility Research Laboratory, Chaim Sheba Medical Center (Tel Hashomer), Ramat Gan, Israel*
SILVINA EPSZTEJN-LITMAN • *Stem Cell Research Laboratory, Medical Genetics Institute, Shaare Zedek Medical Center, Jerusalem, Israel*
MORAN FRIEDMAN GOHAS • *The Fertility Research Laboratory, Chaim Sheba Medical Center (Tel Hashomer), Ramat Gan, Israel*
BRUCE E. HAYWARD • *Section on Gene Structure and Disease, Laboratory of Cell and Molecular Biology, National Institute of Diabetes, Digestive and Kidney Diseases, National Institutes of Health, Bethesda, MD, USA*
JACK FARO VANDER STOEP HUNT • *Waisman Center, University of Wisconsin-Madison, Madison, WI, USA*
PENG JIN • *Department of Human Genetics, Emory University School of Medicine, Atlanta, GA, USA*
SIMON D. KLAPPER • *Center for Regenerative Therapies, Technische Universität Dresden, Dresden, Germany*
HA EUN KONG • *Department of Human Genetics, Emory University School of Medicine, Atlanta, GA, USA*
RUTH KORNREICH • *Department of Genetics and Genomic Sciences, Icahn School of Medicine at Mount Sinai, New York, NY, USA; Sema4, a Mount Sinai Venture, Stamford, CT, USA*

LISA K. KUTSCHE • *Center for Regenerative Therapies, Technische Universität Dresden, Dresden, Germany*
LIRON KUZNITSOV-YANOVSKY • *Wolfe PGD Stem Cell Lab, Racine IVF Unit at Lis Maternity Hospital, Tel Aviv Sourasky Medical Center, Tel Aviv, Israel; Department of Cell and Developmental Biology, Sackler Faculty of Medicine, Tel Aviv University, Tel Aviv, Israel*
MENG LI • *Waisman Center, University of Wisconsin-Madison, Madison, WI, USA*
JUNGHWA LIM • *Department of Human Genetics, Emory University School of Medicine, Atlanta, GA, USA*
YOAV MAYSHAR • *Wolfe PGD Stem Cell Lab, Racine IVF Unit at Lis Maternity Hospital, Tel Aviv Sourasky Medical Center, Tel Aviv University, Tel Aviv, Israel*
ULLA-KAISA PETERI • *Faculty of Medicine, Physiology, University of Helsinki, Helsinki, Finland*
ADI RECHES • *Genetic Institute and Racine IVF Unit at Lis Maternity Hospital Tel Aviv, Sackler Faculty of Medicine, Tel Aviv Sourasky Medical Center, Tel Aviv University, Tel Aviv, Israel*
EVELYN J. SAUTER • *Center for Regenerative Therapies, Technische Universität Dresden, Dresden, Germany*
MENAHEM SEGAL • *Department of Neurobiology, The Weizmann Institute of Science, Rehovot, Israel*
FLORA TASSONE • *Department of Biochemistry and Molecular Medicine, University of California Davis School of Medicine, Davis, CA, USA; MIND Institute, University of California Davis Medical Center, Sacramento, CA, USA*
MICHAEL TELIAS • *Department of Molecular and Cell Biology, University of California, Berkeley, CA, USA*
KAREN USDIN • *Section on Gene Structure and Disease, Laboratory of Cell and Molecular Biology, National Institute of Diabetes, Digestive and Kidney Diseases, National Institutes of Health, Bethesda, MD, USA*
IRENA VERTKIN • *Department of Cell and Developmental Biology, Tel Aviv Sourasky Medical Center, Tel Aviv University, Tel Aviv, Israel*
HAOLEI WAN • *Department of Genetics and Genomic Sciences, Icahn School of Medicine at Mount Sinai, New York, NY, USA; Sema4, a Mount Sinai Venture, Stamford, CT, USA*
MARWA ZAFARULLAH • *Department of Biochemistry and Molecular Medicine, University of California Davis School of Medicine, Davis, CA, USA*
XINYU ZHAO • *Waisman Center, University of Wisconsin-Madison, Madison, WI, USA; Department of Neuroscience, University of Wisconsin-Madison, Madison, WI, USA*

Part I

FXS: Full Mutation

Chapter 1

Fragile X Syndrome: Introduction

Adi Reches

Abstract

Fragile X syndrome (FXS) is one of the most common reasons for intellectual disability (ID). First described in the 1940s, it took many years to understand the disease. The awe-inspiring breakthroughs in both science and technology facilitated the recognition of the unique inheritance pattern and the genetic mechanism of fragile X. In this chapter we describe the history and evolution of our understanding of FXS as mirrored by advances in genetics.

Key words Martin JP, Bell J, Lubs HA, Inheritance pattern, Sherman paradox, Premutation, Trinucleotide repeats expansions, Anticipation, *FMR1* gene, Testing for fragile X syndrome, Clinical features of FXS, Fragile X-associated tremor/ataxia syndrome, Primary ovarian insufficiency, Prenatal diagnosis

1 Historical Background

Fragile X syndrome (FXS) is the second most common reason for intellectual disability (ID), after trisomy 21 and the first cause of inherited ID. It was first defined in 1943 by Martin and Bell, describing a large pedigree of an extensive family which they followed for over 17 years, in which 11 male members born to mothers described as healthy had ID. They also described more mildly affected female members of the extended family. This was the first report of an X-linked inheritance pattern of ID [1].

In 1969, Lubs first reported a distinct chromosomal finding which was termed a "marker chromosome with secondary constriction" on the X chromosome that segregated with ID in three generations of a family [2]. Further testing of males elucidated a fragile site near the distal portion of the long arm of the X chromosome. At metaphase the two chromatids appear to be thinned to a thread—such thinning of the chromatin is termed a fragile site, hence the term "Fragile X." Special culture conditions were needed and the diagnosis was technically challenging. Consequently the fragile site was sublocalized by high-resolution microscopy to band Xq27.3 and FXS defined as a clinical and cytogenetic entity [3].

Dalit Ben-Yosef and Yoav Mayshar (eds.), *Fragile-X Syndrome: Methods and Protocols*, Methods in Molecular Biology, vol. 1942, https://doi.org/10.1007/978-1-4939-9080-1_1,

Still, the disease continued to puzzle as to the exact inheritance pattern. At first, it was believed that FXS was an X-linked recessive genetic disorder. However, the clinical data observed was inconsistent with this. If the disorder was truly inherited in an X-linked recessive manner, heterozygote women should not display any characteristics of the syndrome, and all carrier males should. Nevertheless, males who were obligate carriers, appeared to be nonpenetrant with no physical or mental features of the syndrome and no expression of the on cytogenetic analysis. However, these "normal transmitting males" passed on their X chromosome to all their daughters, who were nonexpressing carriers as well but who then had affected sons. The daughter of an unaffected male carrier was more likely to have affected offspring than the mother of the unaffected male carrier was. This observation became known as the "Sherman paradox." Moreover, there were reports of affected females. What mode of inheritance could reconcile that some male carriers could be so severely affected while others were completely unaffected? [4]. It seems as though there must be some novel genetic mechanisms operating at the fragile X locus to explain this remarkable inheritance pattern [5].

One possible hypothesis given was that the assumed gene for FXS was mutated in a two-step process. The first mutation caused a "premutation" state that produced no clinical symptoms, and a later second mutation was required to convert the premutation to a "full mutation" form that was associated with the characteristic symptoms of FXS. Furthermore, the conversion from a premutation to a full mutation was propositioned to occur only when the premutation was transmitted from a carrier female to her offspring. This theory would take several years to be proven.

It was only in 1991 that an international team of scientists identified the gene and mutation that causes FXS. They found that in families with FXS, there is an untranslated portion of exon 1, upstream to the translational start (5′) with an expanded length of CGG trinucleotide repeats [6]. It was discovered that in males with the clinical phenotype of the FXS, the FMR protein was absent, most likely as a result of transcriptional silencing of the corresponding *FMR1* gene [7]. This silencing occurs as a consequence of the expansion of the number of repeats of the trinucleotide CGG in the 5′ untranslated region (UTR) of the gene.

FXS was discovered to result from an expanded length in a CGG repeat area found in the coding sequence of the *FMR1* gene. Normal individuals analyzed had a low number of repeats, classified initially with 6 to 54 repeats. Obligate premutation carriers in fragile X families without any initial phenotypic effect were found to carry repeats ranging in size from 52 to over 200 repeats. Alleles with greater than 52–55 repeats (premutation alleles) were considered meiotically unstable. They were termed a premutation state because the number of repeats was not sufficient to cause

ID. This range of repeats may predispose to other disorders as discussed later. Those with 46 repeats and lower were considered stable. The Sherman paradox was resolved: the risk of expansion during oogenesis to the full mutation associated with mental retardation increases with the number of repeats [8]. Over the years the criteria for premutation carriers have been revised.

Additional molecular studies identified a stepwise amplification of the trinucleotide CGG repeat element within the 5′ of the FMR1 gene on the fragile X chromosome. With further amplification, this CGG area expands noticeably and as a result the FMR1 gene promoter becomes highly methylated and gene activity is lost [9]. An expansion of more than 200 repeats termed "full mutation" and is accompanied by abnormal methylation on the active X chromosome and is clinically associated with fragile X mental retardation (FXMR) [10]. Identification of a male with the typical characteristics of the FXS, without the characteristic expansion in the FMR1 gene, but rather a de novo microdeletion of the proximal part of this gene, was an additional indication that the *FMR1* gene is truly responsible for the clinical features of the syndrome [11].

In view of the low reproductive fitness of affected males, the high incidence of the syndrome was first suggested to result from a high rate of new mutations in the male germ line. However, family studies failed to identify cases of a new mutation. Rather, carriers and affected individuals alike were found to have inherited the mutation from a parent also carrying an expanded allele. It was postulated that alleles of over 50 copies of CGG arise from normal alleles, but these are nonphenotypic and stable for many generations. This longevity allows the necessary time for the establishment of an ancestral haplotype. It was proposed that these larger CGG alleles convert to premutations at a frequency of 1%–2% per generation. They are then highly unstable and progress rapidly to a full fragile X mutation. This rapid expansion accounts for the high mutation rate observed in family studies. Hence, a pool of preexisting, or predisposed carriers constantly gives rise to new fragile X cases [12, 13].

The identification of FMR1 and the expanded CGG repeats was a landmark discovery in human genetics because it established a novel class of human genetic mutations, trinucleotide (or triplet) repeat expansions. Since the discovery of FMR1 and the expanding CGG repeats, scientists have identified more than ten other human genetic disorders that are caused by expansions of trinucleotide repeats, including disorders such as Huntington's disease and Myotonic Dystrophy.

FMR1 is widely expressed in both human and mouse embryos, with the highest expression located in the brain, testes, ovaries, esophageal epithelium, thymus, eye, and spleen [14]. The fragile X mental retardation protein (FMRP) is the protein product of *FMR1*. FMRP contains two ribonucleoprotein K homology domains (KH domains) and clusters of arginine and glycine residues (RGG boxes), two features commonly associated with RNA-binding proteins [15]. The FMRP is primarily a cytoplasmic protein, but it has also been localized in the neuronal nucleoplasm and within the nuclear pore [16]. It is involved in the regulation of post-transcriptional RNA metabolism and plays an important role in synaptic plasticity, dendrite and axon development, and thus underlying learning and memory. FMRP acts as an organizer of both mRNA transport (shuttle protein), targets mRNA translation (RNA-binding protein) and is involved in a feedback loop by controlling its own local protein levels [17].

Testing for FXS has evolved over time. Analysis of the historical fragile site was soon discontinued as a diagnostic method. The gold standard for many years was the Southern blot, used with or without methylation status. However, neither of these measures could be used to predict the degree of mental retardation status for either sex [18]. The main disadvantage of the Southern blot is that it requires a large amount of DNA and is rather laborious. Both these features encumbered the rapid and inexpensive screening of large populations. Due to these limitations, other diagnostic tests based on the DNA and protein properties of the FXS were developed over the years. PCR-based protocols with different degrees of amplification abilities and sizing accuracies were utilized. Their main advantages were speed, automation, low cost, and the small amount of DNA needed. But the test results were not always straightforward. It is not possible to tell the difference between a female who is homozygous for a normal allele and one who has a large nonamplifiable second allele. Similarly, patients who are mosaics for premutations and full mutations will appear to have only premutations. Moreover, it could only reveal alleles with up to ~300 repeats in males and up to ~160 repeats in females and it therefore fails to identify the large CGG expansions (e.g., more than 300 CGGs). To avoid these false negatives, many screening programs continued to utilize Southern Blot as a follow-up method for samples that failed to amplify by PCR or for females that appeared to be homozygous [19]. The limitations of the PCR plus southern Blot technique lead to the development of new PCR-based procedures able to detect all FMR1 alleles. Triplet primed PCR (TP-PCR) AGG trinucleotide repeat is a procedure in which the CGG repeat number is determined by fragment sizing of PCR amplicons using capillary electrophoresis [20]. This technique allows for the simultaneous amplification of both the full-length FMR1 alleles and CGG triplets in the same PCR reaction and is now the gold standard for the first level assessment of FXS and can detect the expanded allele even when in a mosaic fashion. In stable normal alleles the CGG region is interrupted by an AGG triplet after every 9/10 CGG repeats. Premutation alleles have fewer AGG interruptions compared with normal-size FMR1 alleles.

These AGG triplets are thought to anchor the region during replication and prevent strand slippage, probably essential for stability of the CGG repeats. This analysis also determines the number and location of AGG trinucleotide interruptions within the tract of CGG repeats of *FMR1*. The number and position of AGG trinucleotide repeats are known to be important in the overall stability of the CGG repeat sequence. Recent results have linked the length of the uninterrupted 3′CGG repeat length with expansion and suggest a minimum threshold for expansion risk [21].

2 Clinical Features of FXS

Males with a full mutation: Males with a full mutation always exhibit some symptoms of the disorder and will be affected. They typically show significant intellectual disability and delayed motor and speech developmental milestones. They have a particular facial appearance characterized by a large head size, a long face, prominent forehead and chin, and protruding ears. In addition males who have FXS have macroorchidism—large testes postpubertal. There is a greater predisposition to behavioral problems such as hyperactivity, hand flapping and hand biting, social anxiety, and temper tantrums. Connective tissue problems may include ear infections, flat feet, high arched palate, double-jointed fingers, and hyperflexible joints. Many of them are also diagnosed with autistic spectrum disorder. They often display poor eye contact, perseverative speech, problems in impulse control and distractibility. Physical problems that are associated with the syndrome include strabismus, mitral valve prolapse, aortic root dilatation, and occasional dermatological problems.

Females heterozygous for the full-mutation alleles: The physical and behavioral features seen in males with FXS have been reported in females heterozygous for the full mutation. Approximately 50% of females who have a full *FMR1* mutation are intellectually disabled; however, they are usually less severely affected than males with a full mutation. The variability among females is believed to result from the ratio in the brain of active X chromosomes with the *FMR1* full mutation to inactive X chromosomes with the normal *FMR1* allele.

Premutation carriers: Males and females who have a fragile X premutation have normal intellect and appearance. Nonetheless, a few individuals both male and female with nondebilitating minor manifestations of FXS have been reported, with including subtle intellectual or behavioral symptoms such as learning difficulties or social anxiety [22].

Fragile X-associated tremor/ataxia syndrome (FXTAS) is characterized by late-onset progressive cerebellar ataxia and intention tremor in persons who are premutation carriers [23]. Other neurologic manifestations are short-term memory loss, cognitive decline, parkinsonism and dementia, peripheral neuropathy, and proximal muscle weakness [24]. Both males and females carriers are at increased risk for FXTAS. The penetrance is age related and is estimated at 40%–45% for carrier males older than 50 years. FXTAS is more difficult to ascertain in females because of milder clinical presentation. Penetrance is also much lower in females (16.5%) [25]. Studies indicate that a correlation exists between repeat lengths and the increasing likelihood of developing FXTAS as do neuroradiologic signs [26].

FMR1-related primary ovarian insufficiency (POI)—Female premutation carriers are at risk for premature ovarian insufficiency—POI. Premature ovarian insufficiency (POI) is defined as cessation of menses before age 40. Currently, no consensus exists for estimating an absolute risk for POI when a woman has high normal or intermediate repeat alleles. Several studies have estimated to be 15%–27% in premutation carriers, compared to a 1% background risk [27, 28]. Surprisingly, however, this relationship is nonlinear. Indeed, the risk appears to increase with increasing premutation repeat size between 59 and 99, thereafter the risk of premature ovarian failure plateaus or even decreases for women with repeat sizes over 100 [29]. Women with full-mutation alleles are not at increased risk for POI.

3 Prenatal Diagnosis and Preimplantation Genetic Diagnosis

Women carriers of a premutation or a full mutation are at risk for an affected offspring. Their reproductive choices include prenatal diagnosis by chorionic villus sampling (CVS) or amniocentesis, and then the option of termination of an affected pregnancy. This is clinically available for many years [30]. Conversely, they may opt for Preimplantation Genetic Diagnosis (PGD), where an IVF embryo is diagnosed prior to its transfer to the womb so that only embryos free of the full mutation or premutation are returned. This is done via polymorphic DNA markers linked to FMR1 gene and haplotyping, and not by direct diagnosis of the number or repeats [31, 32].

References

1. Martin JP, Bell J (1943) A pedigree of mental defect showing sex-linkage. J Neurol Psychiatry 6(3–4):154–157
2. Lubs HA (1969) A marker X chromosome. Am J Hum Genet 21(3):231–244
3. Krawczun MS, Jenkins EC, Brown WT (1985) Analysis of the fragile-X chromosome: localization and detection of the fragile site in high resolution preparations. Hum Genet 69:209–211
4. Sherman SL, Jacobs PA, Morton NE, Froster-Iskenius U, Howard-Peebles PN, Nielsen KB, Partington MW et al (1985) Further segregation analysis of the fragile X syndrome with special reference to transmitting males. Hum Genet 69:289–299

5. Winter RM (1989) Fragile X mental retardation. Arch Dis Child 64(9):1223–1224
6. Verkerk AJ, Pieretti M, Sutcliffe JS, Fu YH, Kuhl DP, Pizzuti A, Reiner O, Richards S, Victoria MF, Zhang F, Eussen BE, van Ommen GJB, Blonden LAJ, Riggins GJ, Chastain JL, Kunst CB, Galjaard H, Caskey CT, Nelson DL, Oostra BA, Warren ST (1991) Identification of a gene (FMR-1) containing a CGG repeat coincident with a breakpoint cluster region exhibiting length variation in fragile X syndrome. Cell 65(5):905–914
7. Pieretti M, Zhang FP, Fu YH, Warren ST, Oostra BA, Caskey CT, Nelson DL (1991) Absence of expression of the FMR-1 gene in fragile X syndrome. Cell 66(4):817–822
8. YH F, Kuhl DP, Pizzuti A, Pieretti M, Sutcliffe JS, Richards S, Verkerk AJ, Holden JJ, Fenwick RG Jr, Warren ST et al (1991) Variation of the CGG repeat at the fragile X site results in genetic instability: resolution of the Sherman paradox. Cell 67(6):1047–1058
9. Knight S, Hirst MC, Roche A et al (1992) Molecular studies of the fragile X syndrome. Am J Med Genet 43:217–223
10. Rousseau F, Heitz D, Biancalana V, Blumenfeld S, Kretz C, Boué J et al (1991) Direct diagnosis by DNA analysis of the fragile X syndrome of mental retardation. N Engl J Med 325:1673–1681
11. Worhle D, Kotzot D, Hirst M et al (1992) Microdeletion of less than 250 kb including the proximal part of the FMR-I gene and the fragile site, in a male with clinical phenotype of fragile X syndrome. Am J Hum Genet 51:299–306
12. Hirst MC, Knight SJ, Christodoulou Z, Grewal PK, Fryns JP, Davies KE (1993) Origins of the fragile X syndrome mutation. J Med Genet 30(8):647–650
13. Snow K, Tester DJ, Kruckeberg KE, Schaid DJ, Thibodeau SN (1994) Sequence analysis of the fragile X trinucleotide repeat: implications for the origin of the fragile X mutation. Hum Mol Genet 3(9):1543–1551
14. Hinds HL, Ashley CT, Sutcliffe JS, Nelson DL, Warren ST, Housman DE, Schalling M (1993) Tissue specific expression of FMR-1 provides evidence for a functional role in fragile X syndrome. Nature Genet 3:36–43
15. Siomi H, Siomi MC, Nussbaum RL, Dreyfuss G (1993) The protein product of the fragile X gene, *FMR1*, has characteristics of an RNA-binding protein. Cell 74:291–298
16. Feng Y, Gutekunst CA, Eberhart DE, Yi H, Warren ST, Hersch SM (1997) Fragile X mental retardation protein: nucleocytoplasmic shuttling and association with somatodendritic ribosomes. J Neurosci 17:1539–1547
17. Noto v HC, Walsh D, Marron K (2016) The impact of FMR1 gene mutations on human reproduction and development: a systematic review. J Assit Reprod Genet 33 (9):1135–1147
18. Maddalena A, Richards CS, McGinniss MJ, Brothman A, Desnick RJ, Grier RE, Hirsch B, Jacky P, McDowell GA, Popovich B, Watson M, Wolff DJ (2001) Technical standards and guidelines for fragile X: the first of a series of disease-specific supplements to the standards and guidelines for Clinical Genetics Laboratories of the American College of Medical Genetics. Genet Med 3:200–205
19. Crawford DC, Acuna JM, Sherman SL (2001) FMR1 and the fragile X syndrome: human genome epidemiology review. Genet Med 3:359–371
20. Chen L, Hadd A, Sah S, Filipovic-Sadic S, Krosting J, Sekinger E, Pan R, Hagerman PJ, Stenzel TT, Tassone F, Latham GJ (2010) An information-rich CGG repeat primed PCR that detects the full range of fragile X expanded alleles and minimizes the need for southern blot analysis. J Mol Diagn 12:589–600
21. Nolin SL, Glicksman A, Ding X, Ersalesi N, Brown WT, Sherman SL, Dobkin C (2011) Fragile X analysis of 1112 prenatal samples from 1991 to 2010. Prenat Diagn 31:925–931
22. Bourgeois JA, Coffey SM, Rivera SM, Hessl D, Gane LW, Tassone F, Greco C, Finucane B, Nelson L, Berry-Kravis E, Grigsby J, Hagerman PJ, Hagerman RJ (2009) A review of fragile X premutation disorders: expanding the psychiatric perspective. J Clin Psychiatry 70:852–862
23. Jacquemont S, Hagerman RJ, Leehey MA, Hall DA, Levine RA, Brunberg JA, Zhang L, Jardini T, Gane LW, Harris SW, Herman K, Grigsby J, Greco CM, Berry-Kravis E, Tassone F, Hagerman PJ (2004) Penetrance of the fragile X-associated tremor/ataxia syndrome in a premutation carrier population. JAMA 291:460–469
24. Jacquemont S, Leehey MA, Hagerman RJ, Beckett LA, Hagerman PJ (2006) Size bias of fragile X premutation alleles in late-onset movement disorders. J Med Genet 43:804–809
25. Rodriguez-Revenga L, Madrigal I, Pagonabarraga J, Xunclà M, Badenas C, Kulisevsky J, Gomez B, Milà M (2009) Penetrance of FMR1 premutation associated pathologies in fragile X syndrome families. Eur J Hum Genet 17:1359–1362

26. Tassone F, Adams J, Berry-Kravis EM, Cohen SS, Brusco A, Leehey MA, Li L, Hagerman RJ, Hagerman PJ (2007) CGG repeat length correlates with age of onset of motor signs of the fragile X-associated tremor/ataxia syndrome (FXTAS). Am J Med Genet B Neuropsychiatr Genet 144B:566–569
27. Sherman S (2005) Clinical implications of gray-zone FMR1 alleles. American College of Medical Genetics Meeting, Dallas, TX, Abstract #308
28. Wittenberger M, Hagerman R, Sherman S et al (2007) The FMR1 premutation and reproduction. Fertil Steril 87:456–465
29. Ennis S, Ward D, Murray A (2006) Nonlinear association between CGG repeat number and age of menopause in FMR1 premutation carriers. Eur J Hum Genet 14:253–255
30. McKinley MJ, Nicolaides KH, Kearney LU, Heron O (1987) Fragile X syndrome. Br Med J (Clin Res Ed) 295(6603):922
31. Malcov M, Naiman T, Yosef DB, Carmon A, Mey-Raz N, Amit A, Vagman I, Yaron Y (2007) Preimplantation genetic diagnosis for fragile X syndrome using multiplex nested PCR. Reprod Biomed Online 14:515–521
32. Reches A, Malcov M, Ben-Yosef D, Azem F, Amit A, Yaron Y (2009) Preimplantation genetic diagnosis for fragile X syndrome: is there increased transmission of abnormal FMR1 alleles among female heterozygotes? Prenat Diagn 29:57–61

Chapter 2

Clinical Genetic Testing for Fragile X Syndrome by Polymerase Chain Reaction Amplification and Southern Blot Analyses

Xiaoqiang Cai, Mohammad Arif, Haolei Wan, Ruth Kornreich, and Lisa J. Edelmann

Abstract

Fragile X syndrome (FXS) is characterized by mental retardation and in the vast majority of cases it is caused by expansion of CGG trinucleotide repeats in the 5′ untranslated region (or UTR) in the *FMR1* gene on the X chromosome. The size and methylation status of CGG repeats are correlated with the clinical phenotype of *FMR1*-related disorders. The methods used for clinical genetic testing of FXS include polymerase chain reaction (PCR) amplification and Southern blot analyses, which effectively detect alleles with repeats in the normal, intermediate, premutation, and full mutation size ranges, as well as the methylation status of *FMR1* promoter region.

Keywords Fragile X syndrome, *FMR1*, CGG repeat, Triplet repeat-primed PCR, Methylation PCR, Southern blot

1 Introduction

Fragile X syndrome (FXS) is an X-linked genetic disorder characterized by moderate to severe mental retardation with typical facial features [1]. It affects about 1 in 4000 males and 1 in 8000 females, making it the most common form of inherited mental retardation [2]. Mutations in the *FMR1* gene are associated with fragile X syndrome and related disorders. In nearly all (>99%) cases, it is caused by expansion of the trinucleotide repeat CGG in the 5′ untranslated region of the first exon of the *FMR1* gene [3, 4]. The normal size range is considered to be up to 44 copies of the repeat. An intermediate size range exists for alleles of 45–54 repeats, in which some alleles are stable and some are unstable. In some individuals, the number of trinucleotide repeat units is increased to between 55 and 200, and it is known as a premutation. Premutation allele carriers are at increased risk for Fragile

Dalit Ben-Yosef and Yoav Mayshar (eds.), *Fragile-X Syndrome: Methods and Protocols*, Methods in Molecular Biology, vol. 1942, https://doi.org/10.1007/978-1-4939-9080-1_2,

X-associated tremor/ataxia syndrome (FXTAS) and primary ovarian insufficiency (POI). Females carrying a premutation are at risk for their allele to expand to a full mutation (>200 repeats). The chance of expansion to a full mutation increases with the size of the allele. Full mutations contain many hundreds to thousands of copies of the repeat which results in FXS clinical phenotypes [1, 3]. Methylation is typically present on full mutation alleles, except for chorionic villus sampling (CVS) of which the methylation pattern is not yet fully established.

Several methodologies are in use to effectively determine the size of CGG repeats and methylation status of the *FMR1* allele in clinical laboratories. Triplet repeat-primed polymerase chain reaction (PCR) amplification is a novel, single-tube PCR technology. It is designed with two gene-specific primers that flank the triplet repeat region, as well as a third primer that is complementary to the CGG repeats [5–10]. With these three primers, both full-length PCR products and multiple partial PCR products differing by one CGG repeat will be amplified and detected. This method provides robust detection of expanded alleles in both premutation and full mutation ranges and helps to resolve allele zygosity. Detection of methylation status of *FMR1* allele has also been described by modified PCR methods using bisulfie treatment and amplification-specific primers [11, 12]. Another approach to detect methylation status is by using PCR followed by methylation-sensitive restriction enzyme digestion of genomic DNA. This method will accurately determine the methylation fraction for each *FMR1* allele at high resolution, and detects low abundance mosaic alleles with increased sensitivity [13, 14]. Southern blot analysis with either radioactive probes [15–17] or nonradioactive chemiluminescent probes [18] is performed for diagnostic testing or when the premutations and full mutations are detected. These assays are used for carrier screening of females, prenatal diagnosis for at-risk pregnancies, and postnatal diagnosis of *FMR1*-related disorders. Here, we describe detailed procedures of abovementioned methods used in our laboratory for clinical genetic testing for FXS, and include distinctive cases for results interpretation.

2 Materials

All solutions are prepared by using ultrapure water (purifying deionized water, to attain a sensitivity of 18 MΩ-cm at 25 °C) and analytical grade reagents. All reagents are prepared at room temperature (unless indicated otherwise).

2.1 Triplet Repeat-Primed PCR and Methylation PCR (mPCR) Reagents

1. PCR primers: Human *FMR1* F,R Primers, *FMR1* CGG Primer (Asuragen).
2. PCR reagents: GC-Rich AMP Buffer, GC-Rich Polymerase Mix, Diluent (Asuragen).
3. Capillary electrophoresis reagents: Hi-Di Formamide, ROX 1000 Size Ladder (Asuragen).
4. DNA digestion reagents: control enzyme (FAM), digestion enzyme (HEX), digestion buffer and DNA control (Asuragen).
5. mPCR primers: FAM- and HEX-Primers (Asuragen).
6. Process Controls: Purified DNA from either cell lines obtained from Coriell Cell Repositories (Camden, NJ) [19, 20] or affected patients (positive controls).

2.2 Southern Blot Reagents

1. Agarose gel: 1%, freshly made (Invitrogen).
2. Digoxigenin labeled probe for nonradioactive detection (Gene Link).
3. Low stringent washing buffer (2 L 2× SSC–0.1% SDS): Mix 200 mL 20× SSC (Invitrogen) with 10 mL 20% SDS (Invitrogen) and bring the volume to 2 L with purified water. Mix well before use (*see* **Note 1**).
4. High stringent washing buffer (1 L 0.5× SSC–0.1% SDS): Mix 5 mL 20× SSC (Invitrogen) with 5 mL 20% SDS (Invitrogen) and bring the volume to 1 L with purified water. If there is precipitation, warm the buffer and mix well before use (*see* **Note 1**).
5. Blocking buffer: Prepare fresh 300 mL of Buffer MB for each membrane by adding 30 mL of 10% blocking solution for hybridization (Gene Link) and 30 mL of 10× Maleic acid buffer (Gene Link) to 240 mL of purified water (*see* **Note 1**). This buffer will be used for Subheading 3.3.5.
6. 1× Maleic acid buffer: Mix 40 mL 10× Maleic acid buffer (Gene Link) with 360 mL purified water (*see* **Note 1**). This buffer will be used in Subheading 3.3.5.
7. 1× detection buffer: Mix 30 mL 10× AP detection buffer with 270 mL purified water.
8. 0.25 M HCl: Add 10 mL HCl to 500 mL purified water (*see* **Note 1**).
9. 0.4 M NaOH–0.6 M NaCl: Add 600 mL NaCl with 100 mL NaOH, mix well and bring the volume to 2 L (*see* **Note 1**).

3 Methods

3.1 Triplet Repeat-Primed PCR

3.1.1 PCR Master Mix Setup and Thermal Cycling

1. Genomic DNAs are extracted from blood, saliva or prenatal samples (CVS, amniotic fluid) using standard genomic DNA isolation technology. Cell line DNAs are used as Process Controls. Before PCR, clinical and cell line DNA samples are quantified using a NanoDrop spectrophotometer and diluted to 20 ng/μL with PCR grade water.
2. To a new semi-skirt 96-well plate, add 2 μL of diluted DNA template to each well. For blank samples, add 2 μL water/diluent into the appropriate well. Add 2 μL of each process control to the appropriate wells (*see* **Note 2**).
3. Thaw all reagents except polymerase mix at room temperature for about 10 mins. Keep the polymerase mix on ice. Vortex all reagents except the polymerase mix (*see* **Note 3**).
4. Add reagents to the master mix tube in the exact order listed: 11.45 μL of GC-Rich AMP buffer, 0.5 μL of Human *FMR1* F, R Primers, 0.5 μL of *FMR1* CGG Primer, 0.5 μL of Diluent, and 0.05 μL of GC-Rich Polymerase Mix (*see* **Note 4**).
5. Vortex the tube containing master mix prior to dispensing to ensure adequate mixing of all reagents.
6. Add 13 μL master mix to each reaction well containing 2 μL DNA or water.
7. Seal the plate with an adhesive film seal (*see* **Note 5**).
8. Gently vortex the plate.
9. Centrifuge the plate to remove bubbles (1 min at 1600 rcf at room temperature) (*see* **Note 6**).
10. Samples in the sealed plates amplified with an initial heat denaturation step of 95 °C for 5 mins, followed by 10 cycles of 97 °C for 35 s, 62 °C for 35 s, and 68 °C for 4 mins, and then 20 cycles of 97 °C for 35 s, 62 °C for 35 s, and 68 °C for 4 mins with a 20-s autoextension at each cycle. The final extension step is 72 °C for 10 mins. Proceed to the next step or freeze PCR products at −20 °C until ready to use (*see* **Note** 7).

3.1.2 Capillary Electrophoresis for Fragment Sizing

1. Thaw Hi-Di Formamide and ROX 1000 size standard to room temperature.
2. Prepare master mix with 1 μL ROX 1000 size standard and 5 μL Hi-Di Formamide for each PCR reaction. Vortex and spin down briefly to mix (*see* **Notes 8**).
3. Aliquot 6 μL size standard/Hi-Di mix to each well of the electrophoresis plate.
4. Make a 1:10 dilution of PCR products with PCR grade water.

5. Transfer 1 μL of the diluted PCR product to the electrophoresis plate containing ROX 1000 and Hi-Di.
6. Fill any remaining wells with 7 μL Hi-Di (*see* **Note 9**).
7. Spin down the plate and seal with adhesive film seal.
8. Denature the samples at 95 °C for 2 mins in the thermocycler and incubate the plate on ice for 2 mins. Protect the plate from light and run the plate in the capillary electrophoresis instrument (*see* **Note 10**).
9. Capillary electrophoresis is performed in the Applied Biosystems 3730xl with a 36-cm capillary (using POP-7 polymer). The injection is at 2.5 kV for 20 s and the run is at 15 kV for 40 mins.

3.1.3 Data Analysis and Interpretation

1. Data from the capillary electrophoresis is analyzed by GeneMapper 4.0/4.1 or equivalent software.
2. Copy the data folder for the run(s) to the GeneMapper data folder. Also make a copy of the folder again so there are two copies of the data.
3. Add the data folder from the run and the copy folder to a new project.
4. For each sample select the analysis method, panel, and select the ROX 1000 size standard according to manufacturer's instruction. Highlight the columns and press Ctrl + D to fill the settings into every sample.
5. Click the green arrow to start the sample analysis.
6. Once analyzed, click on the size match editor and confirm that the size standard has been aligned correctly in each sample.
7. Now sort the samples in order of the sample names so that two versions of each sample can be viewed at the same time.
8. Open the two traces for each sample in the plot viewer (Fig. 1a). Confirm the appropriate selection of gene-specific peaks. Peaks can be selected, deselected, and labeled by double-clicking on the peak (*see* **Note 11**).
9. Zoom in on the peaks in each sample as appropriate to ensure that no peaks present are missing.
10. Print a sheet for each sample using large-size output and landscape orientation.
11. Once the appropriate peaks have been selected for each sample and export the genotypes table as .txt files.
12. Open the genotype table with the excel program and copy the data to the Data Analysis Macro excel sheet.

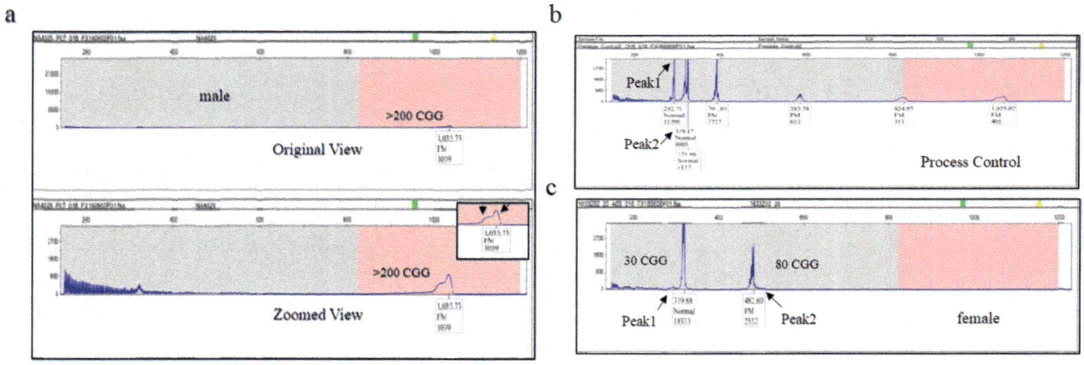

Fig. 1 Fragile X PCR electropherograms. Male full mutation (>200 CGG repeats, Fig. 1a) displayed in both original (upper panel) and zoomed views (lower panel). The highest peak is selected (arrow), whereas other peaks (arrow head) are deselected as shown in inset picture. Electropherograms of process control (Fig. 1b) and female premutation (PM) (Fig. 1c) are shown respectively

13. Copy the sample name and corresponding gender list matched with sample map and paste to the Data Analysis Macro excel sheet.
14. The CGG repeat Allele 1 is calculated by the formula $(size1 - s0)/3 + n0$, Where size1 is equal to the size of the sample's first peak, s0 is equal to the second normal peak of process control, and n0 is equal to allele 2 of process control (Fig. 1b, c).
15. Allele 2 is calculated by the formula $(size2 - s0)/3 + n0$. Where size2 is equal to the size of the sample's second peak, s0 is equal to the second normal peak of process control1, and n0 is equal to allele 2 of process control (Fig. 1b, c).
16. The reportable range is: =<44 = normal, 45--54 = intermediate, 55–200 = premutation (PM), >200 = full mutation (FM).

3.2 Methylation PCR

3.2.1 Genomic DNA Digestion

1. Thaw digestion buffer and DNA control for least 10 mins at room temperature. Place control enzyme (FAM) and digestion enzyme (HEX) on ice.
2. Thoroughly vortex all the tubes (3–5 times pulse vortexing), except the enzymes. Quick spin all the tubes to collect the reagents at the bottom.
3. Measure the absorbance of genomic DNA samples and dilute DNA to 20 ng/μL appropriately with PCR grade water with a total volume of 20 μL.
4. Transfer 8 μL of diluted DNA each to 96-well plate. Add the Process Control in appropriate well of the plate.
5. Add 2 μL of control DNA and vortex well and spin down the plate.

6. Transfer 4 μL of DNA control mix to each of two 96-well plate labeled as FAM-Digestion and HEX-Digestion.
7. Prepare FAM control master mix by adding 3.7 μL digestion buffer and 0.3 μL control enzyme whereas HEX digestion master mix prepared by adding 3.7 μL digestion buffer and 0.3 μL digestion enzyme in separate tubes.
8. Thoroughly vortex master mix (3–5 times pulse vortexing), spin down, and aliquot in 12 strip tubes.
9. Add 4 μL FAM and HEX digestion master mix to each well of corresponding FAM and HEX-Digestion plate separately.
10. Gently vortex reactions and spin down for 10 s (*see* **Note 12**).
11. Incubate at 37 °C for 2 hrs followed by 4 °C hold using thermocycler. When the reaction reaches 4 °C, proceed to methylation PCR within the same day (*see* **Note 13**).

3.2.2 PCR Master Mix Setup and Thermal Cycling

1. Thaw the PCR reagents including mPCR GC-Rich Amp buffer and mPCR FAM- and HEX-Primers at least 10 mins at room temperature. Place GC-Rich Polymerase Mix on ice.
2. Thoroughly vortex all tubes (3–5 times pulse vortexing) except Polymerase Mix. Quick spin all the tubes to collect the reagents at the bottom.
3. To prepare one of each FAM and HEX PCR master mixes in 1.5 mL microfuge tube, add 1.9 μL of FAM and HEX primer, and add 20 μL mPCR GC-Rich Amp Buffer, 0.1 μL GC-Rich Polymerase Mix in the respective tube.
4. Thoroughly vortex master mix (3–5 times pulse vortexing) prior to aliquoting to strip-tubes.
5. For each DNA sample, dispense 22 μL of FAM-PCR master mix to the FAM-Digestion plate and dispense 22 μL of HEX-PCR master mix to the HEX-Digestion plate from enzyme digestion step.
6. Gently vortex both plates and spin down for 10 secs. Seal the plate with an adhesive film seal (*see* **Note 14**).
7. Place plate in a thermocycler. Run the following PCR profile with heated lid: denaturation step of 98 °C for 5 mins, followed by 27 cycles of 97 °C for 35 s, 62 °C for 35 s, and 72 °C for 4 mins, followed by final extension at 72 °C for 10 mins with hold at 4 °C (*see* **Note 15**).

3.2.3 Capillary Electrophoresis for Fragment Sizing

1. Thaw the Hi-Di formamide and ROX 1000 size standard for 10 mins at room temperature. Thoroughly vortex (up to 15 secs) and spin tubes before use.
2. Transfer 5 μL of FAM-PCR products to a new 96-well plate, and then transfer 5 μL of HEX-PCR products to the same plate

with the matching FAM-labeled PCR product (mixed PCR product plate).

3. Transfer 2 μL of mixed PCR product to new capillary electrophoresis analysis plate.
4. Prepare master mix with 2 μL ROX 1000 size standard and 11 μL Hi-Di Formamide for each PCR reaction.
5. Mix all added reagents (by pulse vortexing 3–5 times), and spin down briefly to collect.
6. Transfer 13.0 μL of Hi-Di/size standard solution to each well of a capillary electrophoresis analysis plate (*see* **Note 16**).
7. Vortex and centrifuge at 2000 rpm (805 rcf) for 10–30 secs to remove bubbles, and transfer to a thermocycler.
8. Denature the samples at 95 °C for 2 mins and transfer the plate to ice. Protect the plate from light and run the plate within 12 hrs.
9. The capillary electrophoresis is performed in the Applied Biosystems 3730xl with a 36-cm capillary (using POP-7 running polymer). The injection is carried out at 2.5 kV for 20 secs and the run is carried out at 15 kV for 40 mins.
10. After the run, the data is analyzed for CGG repeat length by amplicon size conversion and for methylation percentage by the ratio of normalized peak heights for each allele PCR product from HEX and FAM channels.

3.2.4 Data Analysis and Interpretation

1. GeneMapper 4.0/4.1 or equivalent software used for fragment sizing analysis of methylation PCR data.
2. Qualify the run by screening the ROX size standard peaks and reviewing Process Controls.
3. Select the peaks in FAM and the matching peaks in the HEX channels. Selection of matching peaks in both the FAM and HEX channels is used for calculating percent methylation (Fig. 2).
4. Genotype tables are exported as .txt files under the table setting established for mPCR Application and uploaded to the Amplidex FMRl mPCR analysis macro according to manufacturer's instruction.
5. The CGG repeat length of the allele peak is converted from base pairs by subtracting the corrected size of the non-CGG repeat region of the amplicon and dividing by the relative size of the CGG repeat region.
6. For each allele in the sample, the methylation percentage is calculated as a ratio of peak heights between the digested

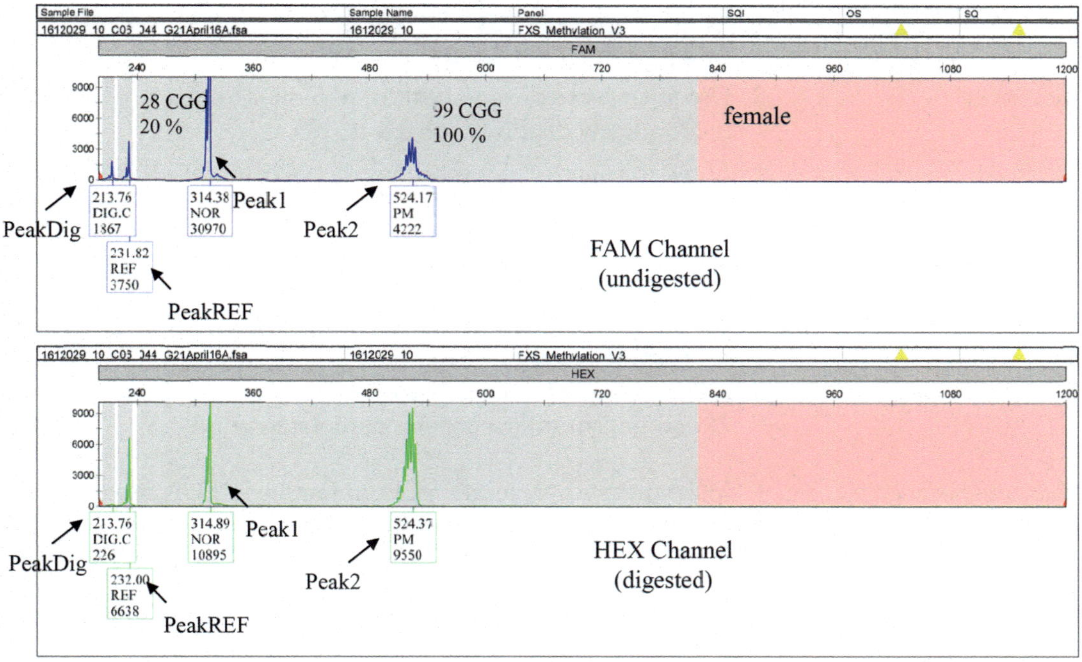

Fig. 2 Electropherogram pattern of Fragile X methylation PCR. After capillary electrophoresis analysis, the electropherograms analyzed from control (FAM) and corresponding digestion (HEX) reaction to identify full length product peaks and the associated percentages. The methylation percentage for each allele determined from the ratio of amplicon peak height in HEX relative to FAM, after normalization by the corresponding CGG control (REF peak) within the same channel

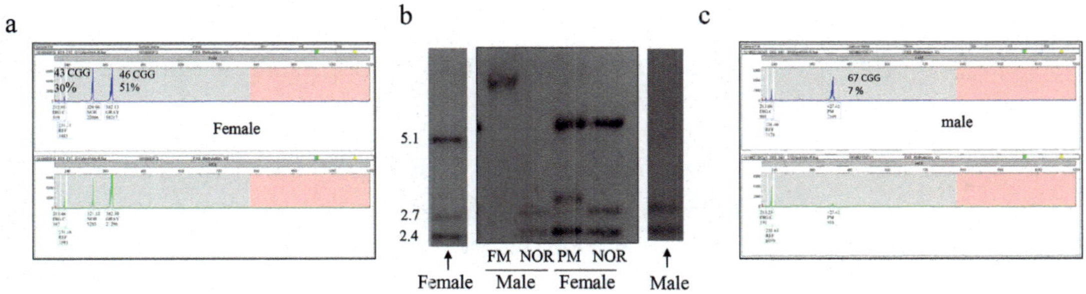

Fig. 3 Fragile X methylation PCR electropherograms and Southern blot images of female and male samples. (**a**) normal female and (**c**) PM male sample (direct chorionic villus, DCV) shown with CGG repeat and corresponding methylation percentage. Southern blot image shown in middle panel (**b**)

(HEX) and undigested samples (FAM) normalized to the CGG control amplicon peak height (*see* **Notes 17–19**).

7. Methylation status reported as <20% = unmethylated, 20%–80% = partially methylated and > 80% = fully methylated (Fig. 3).

3.3 Southern Blot

3.3.1 Prepare 1% Agarose Gel

1. Weigh 6.5 g agarose powder and transfer to a 1 L glass beaker.
2. Add 650 mL 1× TAE and mix well.
3. Use microwave oven to heat for 3–5 mins until agarose powder is completely dissolved (*see* **Note 20**).
4. Allow the agarose gel solution to cool down at room temperature for 5 mins and add 6.5 μL Ethidium Bromide (EB).
5. Pour the agarose gel solution slowly into gel tray (Thermo Scientific Owl wide gel tray) with the 24-well comb (Thermo Scientific) in place. Make sure that there is no visible bubble (*see* **Note 21**).
6. Allow the agarose gel to sit at room temperature for 20–30 mins until it becomes completely solid.

3.3.2 Genomic DNA Digestion and Gel Electrophoresis Separation

1. Make digestion reaction for each sample in PCR tube. Volume of each component: SmartCut NEB buffer 5 μL, Spermidine 5 μL, *EagI* (20 μ/μL) 4 μL, *EcoRI* (100μ/μL) 1 μL, and genomic DNA (5 μg) up to 85 μL. The total volume for each reaction is 100 μL. Make sure to include one positive control and one negative control for each gender (*see* **Note 22**).
2. Use 96-well thermocycler to digest the reaction for 4–16 hrs and then keep the reaction at 4 °C until ready to load the gel.
3. Mix samples with 6μ loading dye and load samples to 1% agarose gel. Load 3 μL 100 bp ladder (Invitrogen) and 5 μL DIG labeled marker (Sigma-Aldrich) on each row of gels.
4. Electrophorese overnight at 45 mA for 16 h. Cut the gel between 1 kb and 3.5 kb to proceed. Take the gels carefully out of the gel tray and put it in the plastic box. Pay attention that you do not mix them up if working on multiple gels (*see* **Note 23**).

3.3.3 DNA Transfer

1. Depurinate with 0.25 M HCl for 10 mins with gentle rotation.
2. Denature the DNA with 0.4 M NaOH–0.6 M NaCl for 30 mins at room temperature with gentle rotation.
3. Rinse the gel with deionized water for 2 mins.
4. Discard the electrophoresis buffer and wipe the tank. Put the electrophoresis tray upside down as a bridge. Put one piece of Whatman paper (GE Life Science 3 MM CHR) on top of the bridge and pour 10× SSC over the bridge with a serological glass pipette to wet thoroughly. Make sure that the paper is soaked in the electrophoresis chambers on both sides with enough 10× SCC buffer.
5. Place gel-well side down on the Whatman paper and remove air bubbles by rolling a serological glass pipette across the gel.

6. Cut the exact size of nylon membrane (Sigma-Aldrich) and label the side facing agarose gel with setup date by pencil. Cut one corner for orientation reference.
7. Dip membrane in 2× SSC buffer and place on gel with labeled side down. Remove air bubbles by using serological glass pipette.
8. Cut two pieces of Whatman paper with same size as gel and place them on top of the nylon membrane. Put one pack of paper towels on top of Whatman paper. Place a water bottle on top for weight.
9. Use Parafilm strips to butt up against the gel on all sides to create a barrier between the bridge and the Whatman paper/paper towels on top.
10. Let the DNA transfer overnight to the nylon membrane.
11. After overnight transfer, approximately half of the paper towels should be soaked with the buffer. Peel the membrane off from agarose gel and place it with labeled side up in a plastic box. Pour 100 mL 2× SSC buffer and allow the membrane to stay for 1 min.
12. Bake the membrane in an 80 °C oven for 2 hrs.

3.3.4 Hybridization

1. Denature 120 μL deoxyribonucleic acid single stranded DNA from salmon testes sperm (Sigma-Aldrich) for 10 mins at 99 °C and cool down on ice immediately for at least 5 mins.
2. Bend the nylon membrane and put it in the hybridization cylinder with date-labeled side facing inward. Mix the denatured DNA with 10 mL of Easy Hyb buffer (Sigma-Aldrich). Add the buffer mixure directly to the bottom of hybridization cylinder by using serological glass pipette.
3. Cap tightly and invert the cylinder multiple times. Balance the cylinder as necessary in the oven and set rotation on speed 7 for at least 3 hrs to perform prehybridization (*see* **Note 24**).
4. Denature 40 μL GeneProber® GLHDDig2× probe (Fragile X CGG Repeat GeneProber, Genelink) in 500 μL of Easy Hyb buffer for 10 mins at 99 °C and then cool down immediately on ice for at least 5 mins.
5. Add the above probe mixture to the bottom of prehybridization cylinder with nylon membrane. Cap tightly and invert the cylinder multiple times. Continue hybridization at the same temperature overnight (*see* **Note 25**).

3.3.5 Washing

1. Wash the membrane in 2× SSC–0.1% SDS in high speed at room temperature twice (15 mins/wash). Make sure that the DNA-labeled side (also the date labeled side) of the membrane face up during washing step (*see* **Note 26**).

2. Use water to rinse the membrane shortly and then wash membrane hardly by 0.1× SSC–0.1% SDS twice at 65 °C (30 mins/wash). Warm the blocking reagent at this point. Make sure that there is no precipitation before use.
3. Wash the membrane in 300 mL of buffer MB (prepared in Subheading 2) in high speed at room temperature for 30 mins.
4. Prepare fresh 300 mL buffer MB for each membrane. Add 30 μL Anti-DIG-AP conjugate solution (Roche Diagnostics) to fresh buffer MB and mix well.
5. Prepare fresh 400 mL 1× buffer Maleic buffer (prepared in Subheading 2). Wash the membrane with 200 mL each time in high speed at room temperature. Repeat one more time wash.
6. Equilibrate the membrane in 100 mL of 1× detection buffer (Genelink) for 5 mins. Repeat 2 times.

3.3.6 Detection

1. Transfer the membrane to the center of a plastic sheet protector and drain off extra buffer. Wipe edges carefully with Kimwipes tissue paper. Keep the membrane wet and proceed quickly.
2. Spray CDP-star ready-to-use substrate (Sigma-Aldrich) evenly to the membrane (*see* **Note 27**). Cover the membrane with plastic sheet protector and wipe the entire surface of the sheet protector to expel any extra substrate and air bubbles.
3. Put membranes (DNA side up) with sheet protector into cassette and go to dark room to put a film on membrane (*see* **Note 28**).
4. Expose film for 1 hr and develop the film with developer machine (*see* **Note 29**).

3.3.7 Blot Stripping

1. Place membrane in a plastic box and wash it with water to remove the substrate.
2. Pour off the water and wash the membrane with 1× stripping buffer (0.2 N NaOH–0.1% SDS) at room temperature for 30 mins.
3. Pour off the stripping buffer and rinse the membrane with 2× SSC.
4. Air-dry the membrane.

3.3.8 Result Interpretation

1. Southern blot analysis for FXS detection involves the cleavage of DNA with enzyme *EcoRI* and *EagI*. This method detects the size of CGG repeats region by hybridization of probe (GLFXDigl GeneProber) to DNA that has been double digested with restriction enzymes *EcoRI* and *EagI* and blotted onto a membrane.

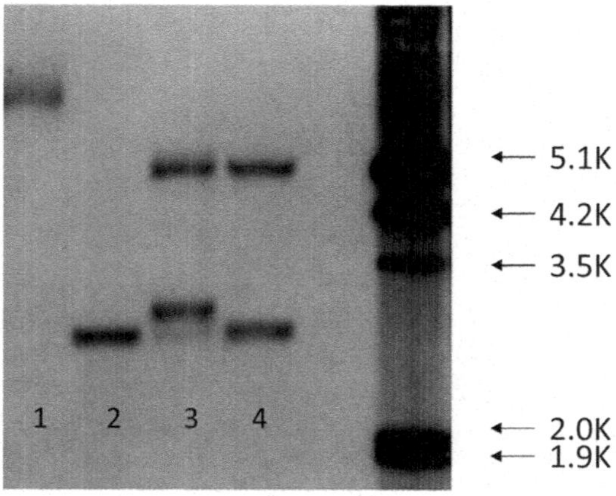

Fig. 4 Lane 1 is a full mutation male with ~645 CGG repeats; Lane 2 is a normal male with 28 repeats; Lane 3 is a premutation female carrier with 30 and 95 repeats, with the larger allele predominantly active; Lane 4 is a normal female with 29 and 31 repeats

2. As shown in Fig. 4, two fragments are seen in normal females. One ~2.8 kb fragment corresponding to the active X chromosome and the other ~5.2 kb fragment corresponding to the methylated inactive X chromosome. Normal males exhibit only the ~2.8 kb fragment. Affected males will have an expanded CGG repeats region with methylation thus giving rise to fragments larger than the normal ~2.8 kb. Premutations in males and females will have fragments from 2.9–3.3 kb (normally 2.8 kb) derived from the active X chromosome. Premutations in females derived from the inactive X will give fragments from 5.3–5.7 kb. Mosaicism is characterized by fragments appearing as a mixture of full mutation (methylated, larger than 5.7 kb) and unmethylated or partially methylated premutation (2.9–3.3 kb) (*see* **Note 30**).

4 Notes

1. The volume is sufficient for two pieces of agarose gel. If more solution is needed, increase the components proportionally.
2. Positive and negative controls are recommended in every run. Genomic DNA extracted from well-characterized cell lines with premutation (PM) and full mutation (FM) alleles may be used for positive controls. At least one negative control must be included in every run. If the signals obtained for the blank are too high, the entire run is rejected and must be repeated.
3. GC-Rich Polymerase mix should be stored on ice all the time. The GC-Rich Amp Buffer may be occluded or have observable

precipitation when cold. After completely thawing the tube, vortex to ensure mixing.

4. Excess GC-Rich Polymerase Mix may inhibit the reaction. Ensure that there are no additional droplets on the pipette tip prior to dispensing to the master mix.
5. Use roller to ensure that all the wells and plate edges are well sealed.
6. Ensure that all bubbles are removed from the wells looking at the plate against the light.
7. PCR product stability at −20 °C has been found to be up to 30 days.
8. Frequent freeze thaw destroys Hi-Di, therefore, we make small aliquots and store at −20 °C to avoid higher background.
9. It is important to fill the empty wells of the plate used in the run to ensure that no bubble is entered in the capillary system.
10. Samples must be denatured prior to capillary electrophoresis analysis and samples may be run up to 24 hrs after denaturation if it is placed on ice or stored at 4 °C.
11. Select only the component of the peak group containing the highest peak. Deselect other peaks within that group. Identify peak as >200 CGG (Fig. 1a).
12. Accurate pipetting and thorough mixing of each reaction is the key to ensuring appropriate methylation ratios for each allele.
13. Do not store or freeze reactions before proceeding to PCR. Keep both FAM and HEX digestion plate on ice until the PCR master mix is ready.
14. To minimize variability, the FAM and HEX PCR reaction mixtures should be treated (vortexed, centrifuged, etc.) as identically as possible throughout the procedure.
15. The PCR products can be transferred for capillary electrophoresis analysis immediately following amplification. If required, the PCR products can be stored at 4 °C overnight or at −20 °C up to 30 days until analyzed.
16. If running less than the number of samples for any injection group, fill empty wells subject to injection with 15 μL of Hi-Di Formamide.
17. For each sample, the effectiveness of the methylation-sensitive enzyme digestion is reported as the percentage of digestion control being digested. A value of 80–90% or more indicates appropriate performance of the digestion reaction. Otherwise, the sample should be retested.

18. For allele peaks with signal intensity beyond the capillary electrophoresis instrument saturation limit, accurate determination of methylation percentages must be derived from a shorter injection of the sample.
19. For allele peaks with low signal intensity in FAM below the capillary electrophoresis instrument cut-off, the high baseline signal in HEX could result in an artificially inflated methylation percentage.
20. Heating time may vary depending on different microwave oven. But do not overboil the solution, as some of the buffer will evaporate and thus alter the final percentage of agarose in the gel.
21. Two combs can be used for each tray. Push any bubbles from the well comb to the edges of the gel with pipette tips.
22. Maximum volume for each reaction is 100 μL. However, the optimized volume is considered as 50 μL or less, so that it is easier to load samples in agarose gel wells. A total of 5 μg is the optimal DNA amount to start. Lower amounts of starting DNA will lead to a weak signal.
23. After the overnight electrophoresis, loading dye should be close to the bottom of the gel. If working on two pieces of gel, cut the right bottom side with different ends so that they can be differentiated. While moving the gel in the plastic box, do not put it upside down.
24. Prehybridization can be longer but not shorter, as it may lead to film with high background.
25. Do not hybridize with probe more than 18 hrs.
26. Put low stringent washing buffer 2× SSC–0.1% SDS in 60 °C water bath until the precipitation is completely dissolved before use.
27. Do not over spray the membrane.
28. Do not move a film that is already on a membrane. Multiple films may be used to achieve a better image. Luminescence continues for at least 24 hrs and signal intensity remains almost constant during the first few hours. Shorter or longer time exposures can be taken to achieve the desired signal strength.
29. Film should always be in dark before development.
30. This test can be used for prenatal diagnosis using DNA extracted from cells obtained from amniocentesis and CVS.

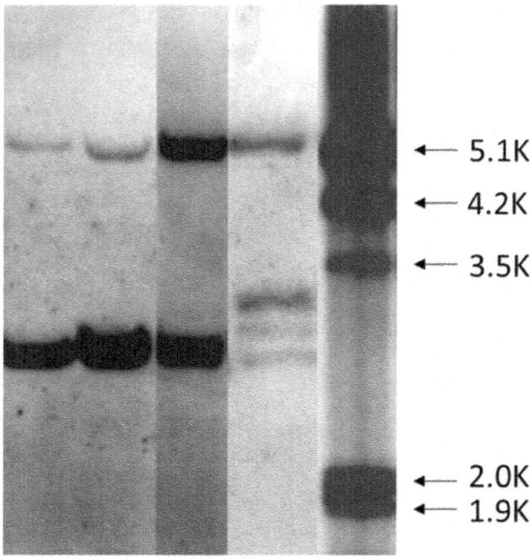

Fig. 5 Lane 1 is a normal prenatal female chorionic villus sample (CVS), and Lane 2 is DNA from a cultured chorionic villus sample from a female fetus with normal repeat sizes. Both samples are not showing an obvious methylation band at ~5.2 kb as compared to a normal female postnatal sample (Lane 3), as methylation is not fully established at the time of CVS. Lane 4 is a mosaic female sample with repeat sizes of approximately 39, 95, 130, and 195

Because methylation is not fully established at the time of CVS, the appearance of full mutations examined by a methylation-specific method may vary in CVS as compared with blood and amniocytes (Fig. 5). Laboratories offering testing of chorionic villi must be aware of this tissue's unique properties.

References

1. Monaghan KG, Lyon E, Spector EB et al (2013) ACMG standards and guidelines for fragile X testing: a revision to the disease-specific supplements to the standards and guidelines for Clinical Genetics Laboratories of the American College of Medical Genetics and Genomics. Genet Med 15(7):575–586
2. Turner G, Webb T, Wake S et al (1996) Prevalence of fragile X syndrome. Am J Med Genet 64(1):196–197
3. Saul RA, Tarleton JC (1998) FMR1-related disorders. GeneReviews. https://www.ncbi.nlm.nih.gov/books/NBK1384/
4. Yu S, Pritchard M, Kremer E et al (1991) Fragile X genotype characterized by an unstable region of DNA. Science 252:1179–1181
5. Tassone F, Pan R et al (2008) A rapid polymerase chain reaction-based screening method for identification of all expanded alleles of the fragile X (FMR1) gene in newborn and high-risk populations. J Mol Diagn 10(1):43–49
6. Chen L, Hadd A et al (2010) An information-rich CGG repeat primed PCR that detects the full range of fragile X expanded alleles and minimizes the need for southern blot analysis. J Mol Diagn 12:589–600
7. Filipovic-Sadic S, Sah S et al (2010) A novel FMR1 PCR method for the routine detection of low abundance expanded alleles and full mutations in fragile X syndrome. Clin Chem 56:399–408
8. Hantash FM, Goos DG et al (2010) Qualitative assessment of FMR1 (CGG)n triplet repeat

status in normal, intermediate, premutation, full mutation, and mosaic carriers in both sexes: implications for fragile X syndrome carrier and newborn screening. Genet Med 12 (3):162–173

9. Lyon E, Laver T et al (2010) A simple, high-throughput assay for fragile X expanded alleles using triple repeat primed PCR and capillary electrophoresis. J Mol Diagn 12(4):505–511
10. Nahhas FA, Monroe TJ et al (2012) Evaluation of the human fragile X mental retardation 1 polymerase chain reaction reagents to amplify the FMR1 gene: testing in a clinical diagnostic laboratory. Genet Test Mol Biomarkers 16 (3):187–192
11. Das S, Kubota T et al (1998) Methylation analysis of the fragile X syndrome by PCR. Genet Test 1(3):151–155
12. Panagopoulos I, Lassen C et al (1999) A methylation PCR approach for detection of fragile X syndrome. Hum Mutat 14(1):71–79
13. Chen L, Hadd A et al (2011) High resolution methylation PCR for fragile X analysis: evidence for novel FMR1 methylation patterns undetected in southern blot analyses. Genet Med 13:528–538
14. Grasso M, Boon EMJ et al (2014) A novel methylation PCR that offers standardized determination of FMR1 methylation and CGG repeat length without southern blot analysis. J Mol Diagn 16:23–31
15. Southern E (2006) Southern blotting. Nat Protoc 1(2):518–525
16. Rousseau F, Heitz D et al (1991) Direct diagnosis by DNA analysis of the fragile X syndrome of mental retardation. N Engl J Med 325(24):1673–1681
17. Nakahori Y, Knight SJ et al (1991) Molecular heterogeneity of the fragile X syndrome. Nucleic Acids Res 19(16):4355–4359
18. Fragile X CGG repeat genotyping GeneProber™ GLFXDig1 manual Catalog No. 40-2004-41
19. Amos Wilson J, Pratt VM et al (2008) Consensus characterization of 16 *FMR1* reference materials: a consortium study. J Mol Diagn 10:2–12
20. Hawkins M, Boyle J et al (2010) Preparation and validation of the first WHO international genetic reference panel for fragile X syndrome. Eur J Hum Genet 19:10–17

Chapter 3

Monitoring for Epigenetic Modifications at the FMR1 Locus

Silvina Epsztejn-Litman and Rachel Eiges

Abstract

The vast majority of fragile X affected patients do not transcribe FMR1 due to a CGG repeat expansion in the 5′-untranslated region of the FMR1 gene. When the CGGs considerably expand, it elicits abnormal DNA methylation and histone modifications, which are responsible for FMR1 transcriptional silencing. In this chapter, we describe in detail two commonly used protocols for monitoring the epigenetic state of the FMR1 gene that bypass the difficulty in directly analyzing the CGGs. One protocol is for accurately measuring DNA methylation levels and the other is for profiling histone modifications.

Key words FMR1, DNA methylation, Histone modifications, Bisulfite DNA sequencing, Chromatin immune-precipitation (ChIP), PCR, qPCR

1 Introduction

The vast majority of fragile X syndrome (FXS) patients carry an unusual loss-of-function mutation due to a CGG trinucleotide microsatellite repeat expansion in the 5′-UTR of the X-linked FMR1 gene [1]. When the CGGs reach the full mutation range (>200 repeats), they lead to incorrect spreading of DNA methylation from the upstream flanking region [2], coupled with a change from active to repressive histone modifications [4–9]. This results in epigenetic gene silencing of FMR1 by a developmentally regulated process, eventually leading to FXS pathology. How precisely the addition of repeats results in the induction of repressive epigenetic marks remains to be elucidated.

Much effort has been invested into developing assays for recording the epigenetic status of the FMR1 gene, particularly for accurate measurement of DNA methylation levels. This is because it may serve as a valuable diagnostic tool for disease prognosis. In addition, it may provide a useful tool for investigating the yet unresolved mechanisms of FMR1 gene silencing in FXS. However, the major difficulties in monitoring the epigenetic changes that are imposed by the mutation lies in the failure to effectively PCR

Dalit Ben-Yosef and Yoav Mayshar (eds.), *Fragile-X Syndrome: Methods and Protocols*, Methods in Molecular Biology, vol. 1942,
https://doi.org/10.1007/978-1-4939-9080-1_3, © Springer Science+Business Media, LLC, part of Springer Nature 2019

amplify the GC-rich repeats, particularly when they are expanded. In this chapter, we describe two commonly used methods for monitoring the epigenetic state of the 5′-end of FMR1 without the need for PCR amplification of the repeats. One method is for accurately measuring DNA methylation levels and the other is for profiling histone modifications (Fig. 1).

Among the currently available tests for monitoring FMR1 DNA methylation (for comprehensive review see Hayward and Usdin [3]), the most sensitive and widely used assay is the one that relies on bisulfite PCR DNA sequencing in the region that is located immediately upstream to the CGGs. The technique is based on chemical pretreatment of DNA with sodium bisulfite, which converts cytosines (Cs) into uracil by deamination, unless they are methylated. First, genomic DNA is denatured and chemically modified by sodium bisulfite, to guarantee efficient C to U conversion. Next, the 5′ or 3′ flanking sequence to the CGGs (a region which is typically methylated when the CGGs expand in cells of patients) is amplified by PCR using a pair of universal strand-specific primers. This permits the simultaneous amplification of methylated (unmodified) and unmethylated (modified) molecules in a single PCR reaction. Finally, the pool of PCR products is sequenced for the identification of C to U conversion events (represented by Ts as a replacement for Cs after PCR amplification), either by single colony Sanger sequencing or locus-specific next-generation sequencing (NGS) (Fig. 1). This provides a convenient way to distinguish between methylated and unmethylated CpG sites at the single molecule level, and it permits analysis of a considerable number of CpG sites simultaneously, at single bp resolution.

For profiling of FMR1 for specific histone modifications in vivo, we use the Chromatin immune-precipitations (ChIP) procedure (Fig. 1). ChIP is a semiquantitative approach that determines whether a given protein–protein posttranscriptional modification binds to a specific DNA sequence in the cell. It is the method of choice for profiling histone modifications, and is commonly used for differentiating transcriptionally active (euchromatin) from inactive chromatin (heterochromatin). The technique is based on the selective enrichment of a chromatin fraction by immunoprecipitation using antibodies that specifically recognize the inspected protein. Briefly, the DNA and the proteins that are associated with chromatin are cross-linked with formaldehyde. Following cell lysis, the DNA is sheared into 250–1000 bp fragments by sonication, and then selectively immunoprecipitated with an antibody that specifically interacts with the targeted protein. Next, the bound DNA fragments are purified from the immunoprecipitated chromatin fraction after cross-linking is reversed. Last, the region of interest is evaluated by qPCR for degree of enrichment by comparing amounts between antibody-immunoprecipitated (bound) and untreated control (input) DNA

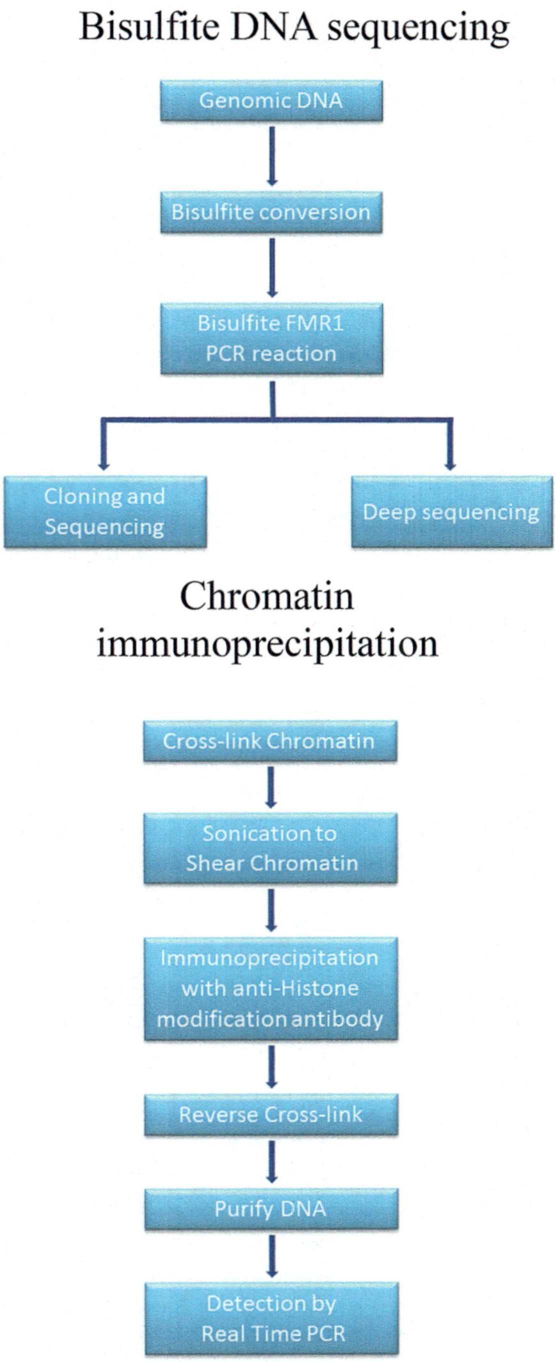

Fig. 1 Workflow

fractions. As ChIP relies on the immunoprecipitation reaction, it is crucial that the antibody will be highly specific and suitable for this type of experimental procedure. In addition, it is absolutely essential to include positive and negative DNA control regions in the analysis. This is to accurately assess the efficiency of the reaction by taking into account the effect of nonspecific signals. One point to consider with respect to FMR1 is that the qPCR reaction, similar to the bisulfite PCR reaction, is carried out by amplification of a region that immediately flanks the CGG sequence. This is to bypass the difficulty of amplifying the CGG repetitive region. However, it should be noted that since enrichments are quantified on sheared DNA fragments (500 bp in average), they provide rough estimates at a resolution of hundreds of bps.

There are by now plenty of commercially available antibodies for carrying out ChIP analysis for the different forms of histone modifications (particularly for the ones that are associated with the silencing of the FMR1 locus) including for histone H3 (K4me3, H3K9me2/3, and H3K27me3) and histone H4 (H4K20me3) [4–9]. For each modification, appropriate positive and negative control amplicons should be selected. This is to validate the efficiency and reliability of the assay.

2 Equipment and Materials

2.1 Bisulfite Reaction

1. Commercially available bisulfite reaction kit, Zymo Bisulfite Direct Kit (#D5020).
2. Eppendorf tubes 1.5 mL and PCR 0.2 μL tubes.
3. Deionized water or TE buffer.
4. PCR thermal cycler.
5. Variable speed centrifuge (benchtop or floor model, >10,000 × *g*).

2.2 PCR Purification, Cloning, and Sequencing Analysis of Target Bisulfite DNA Fragment

1. Fast Start Taq polymerase (Roche).
2. FMR1 gene specific converted primers.

   FMR1 5′ (colony bisulfite):
   Forward 5′-TTGAGTGTATTTTTGTAGAAATGGG-3′.
   Reverse 5′-CCTCTCTCTTCAAATAACCTAAAAA-3′.
   T_m = 55 °C. Product size: 191 bp.
   FMR1 3′ (colony bisulfite):
   Forward 5′-GGTATTTGGTTTTAGGGTAGGTTT-3′.
   Reverse 5'-TTCCAACAAACCCCAAAT-3′.
   T_m = 55 °C. Product size: 173 bp.
3. Agarose gel, ethidium bromide, and electrophoresis apparatus.
4. QIAquick PCR Purification Kit (Qiagen) for purification of PCR product or QIAquick Gel Extraction Kit (Qiagen) for purification of target PCR fragment from multiple nonspecific PCR products.
5. pGEM-T Easy vector system II (Promega).

6. Competent bacteria, DH5α cells.
7. For bacterial culturing and positive cloning selection, Bacto tryptone (BD), yeast extract, sodium chloride, ampicillin solution, isopropyl-β-D-thiogalactoside (IPTG), X-Gal (Bio-Rad), and bacterial shaker incubator at 37 °C are required.
8. Mini prep kit.
9. Colony PCR: Ready mix ×5 (Biolab), SP6 and T7 primers.

2.3 Bisulfite Sanger Sequencing Reaction and Analysis

1. BigDye 3.1 V.
2. PCR thermal cycler.
3. Performa DTR (Dye Terminator Removal) Gel Filtration Cartridges.
4. ABI No# DNA Analyzer.
5. Analysis software Finch TV and ApE-A editor.

2.4 Bisulfite Deep Sequencing

1. Gene-specific primers with P5 or P7 adaptors.

   FMR1 3′ (deep sequencing):
   Forward 5′-P5-AGAGGGGTTTTTAATAGGTTTTAAGTT-3′.
   Reverse 5′-P7-CTTCCCTCCCTTTTCTTCTTAAT-3′.
   $T_m = 55$ °C.
   P5 adaptor: Forward overhang: 5′ TCGTCGGCAGCGTCAG ATGTGTATAAGAGACAG-[locus-specific sequence].
   P7 adaptor: Reverse overhang: 5′ GTCTCGTGGGCTCGG AGATGTGTATAAGAGACAG-[locus-specific sequence]
2. D1000 ScreenTape kit (Agilent Technologies) and Qubit® DNA HS Assay kit (catalog #32854; Invitrogen), (×1, Agencourt AMPure XP—Beckman Coulter.
3. PrimMax Takara taq polymerase and N7XX primer (nextera barcode 1) and S5XX primer (nextera barcode 2), and 2× Primstar)ReadyMix).
4. ScreenTape kit and the Qubit® DNA HS Assay kit for quality control of prepared library and normalization processes.
5. NextSeq 500 Mid-Output Kit (150 cycles) cartridge (Illumina, San Diego, CA) and NextSeq 500 System instrument (Illumina).

2.5 Chromatin Immunoprecipitation Assay Materials

1. E8 supplemented medium (Gibco).
2. Vitronectin.
3. Trypsin.
4. 37% formaldehyde.
5. 1.25 M glycine.
6. 0.5 M EDTA pH 8.0.
7. 5 M NaCl.

8. 1 M Tris–HCl, pH 6.5.
9. 10× PBS.
10. Protease Inhibitor Cocktail II.
11. RNase A.
12. Proteinase K.
13. 1 M $NaHCO_3$.
14. 20% SDS.
15. Antibody of interest for chromatin immunoprecipitation, anti-H3K4me2 (Upstate 07-030), anti-H3K9me3 (Abcam 8898), and anti-H3K27me (Abcam 6002).
16. Protein G magnetic beads.
17. DNA purification kit.
18. SYBR Green mix.
19. Primers:

    HOXA9 Forward 5′-CTCAGGAGCCTCGTGTCTTT-3′.
    Reverse 5′-GTGACCAGGTGGAGGTGTGT-3′.
    T_m = 60 °C, Product Size (bp) = 82.
    CRYSTALIN Forward 5′-CCGTGGTACCAAAGCTGA-3′.
    Reverse 5′-AGCCGGCTGGGGTAGAAG-3′.
    T_m = 58–62 °C, Product Size (bp) = 85.
    APRT Forward 5′-GCCTTGACTCGCACTTTTGT-3′.
    Reverse 5′-TAGGCGCCATCGATTTTAAG-3′.
    T_m = 60 °C, Product Size (bp) = 85.
    FMR1 promoter Forward 5′-AACTGGGATAACCGGATG CAT-3′.

    Reverse 5′-GGCCAGAACGCCCATTTC-3′.
    T_m = 63 °C, Product Size (bp) = 72.
20. DNase- and RNase-free sterile H_2O.
21. SDS Lysis Buffer: 1% SDS, 10 mM EDTA pH 8, 50 mM Tris–HCl pH 8.1.
22. TE buffer 25 mM: 1 mM EDTA pH = 8, 10 mM Tris–HCl pH = 8.
23. Dilution Buffer 10 mL: 1.1.% Triton X-100, 1.2 mM EDTA pH = 8, 16.7 mM Tris–HCl pH = 8, 167 mM NaCl, 8.4 mL DDW.
24. Elution Buffer: 1 mM EDTA pH = 8, 10 mM Tris–HCl pH = 8, 200 mM NaCl, 1% SDS.
25. Low Salt Buffer 25 mL: 1% Triton X-100, 2 mM EDTA pH 8, 20 mM Tris–HCl pH = 8, 150 mM NaCl, 0.1% SDS.
26. High Salt Buffer 25 mL: 1% Triton X-100, 2 mM EDTA pH = 8, 20 mM Tris–HCl pH = 8, 500 mM NaCl, 0.1% SDS.
27. LiCl immune complex wash buffer 25 mL: 1 mM EDTA pH 8, 10 mM Tris–HCl pH 8.1, 1% NP-40, 250 mM LiCl, 1% deoxycholate.

2.6 Chromatin Immunoprecipitation Assay Materials Equipment

1. Biological and chemical hoods.
2. CO_2 incubator.
3. Vortex mixer.
4. Rotating wheel/platform.
5. Timer.
6. Variable volume (5–1000 μL) pipettes + tips.
7. Centrifuge (micro and regular).
8. Variable temperature water bath.
9. Sonicator Bath Vibra Cell VCX130 with 3 mm microtip.
10. Microfuge tubes, 1.5 mL.
11. Real-time PCR.
12. Real-time plates.
13. Filter-tip pipette tips.
14. Electrophoresis equipment.

3 Methods

3.1 Measuring FMR1 Methylation Levels by Bisulfite PCR DNA Sequencing

3.1.1 Bisulfite Conversion

1. Two micrograms of genomic DNA in a total volume of 20 μL DDW is added to 130 μL of CT conversion reagent solution in a PCR tube (EZ DNA Methylation Direct Kit, Zymo). The sample is mixed and centrifuged briefly to ensure that no droplets are in the cap or side of the tube.
2. Place the PCR tube in a thermocycler and perform the following steps:

   98 °C for 8 min.

   64 °C for 3.5 h.

   4 °C storage for up to 20 h.
3. Add 600 μL of M-Binding Buffer into a Zymo-Spin IC column and place the column into a collection tube.
4. Load the sample from **step 2** into the column containing the M-Binding buffer. Close the cap and mix by inverting the column several times.
5. Centrifuge at full speed, ≥10,000 × *g* for 30 s. Discard the flow-through.
6. Add 100 μL of M-wash buffer to the column. Centrifuge at full speed for 30 s.
7. Add 200 μL of M-Desulfonation Buffer to the column and let stand at room temperature (20°–30°) for 15–20 min. After incubation, centrifuge at full speed for 30 s.

8. Add 200 μL of M-wash buffer to the column. Centrifuge at full speed for 30 s. Add another 200 μL of M-Wash buffer and centrifuge for 1 min.
9. Place the column into a 1.5 mL microcentrifuge tube. Add 10 μL of the M Elution Buffer directly to the column matrix. Wait for 1 min and centrifuge for 30 s at full speed to elute the DNA.
10. The DNA is ready for immediate analysis or can be stored at or below −20 °C for later use. For long term storage, store at below −70 °C (*see* **Note 1**).

3.1.2 Bisulfite PCR Amplification

Bisulfite treated DNA can be amplified with strand specific and bisulfite specific primers in a PCR reaction. Primers designed outside of a CpG region of interest will, in principle, amplify the target regardless of the methylation state of the internal sequence. Bisulfite sequencing provides an inherently more accurate assessment of the methylation state of a sample compared to PCR primers (or probes) that select for presupposed fully methylated or fully unmethylated complementary sequences, such as methylation-specific primers (MSP). Bisulfite PCR primer design is crucial for successful implementation of subsequent bisulfite sequencing analysis.

Primer Design

1. Primers have to be ~25–30 bp in length, to ensure specificity.
2. Primer pairs should have a similar Tm, be above 50 °C and not differ by more than 1–2 °C.
3. Primers should contain multiple (~25%) C to T bases, to ensure conversion specificity.
4. The last base at the 3′ end of the primer should be a C to T to ensure amplification of converted DNA.
5. CpGs should be avoided in the primer sequence to circumvent potential bias toward methylated, unmethylated, or unconverted templates.
6. Amplicons length should not be more than ~450 bp (*see* **Note 2**).

Bisulfite PCR Reaction

1. Annealing temperature: A gradient PCR thermocycler can help to determine the appropriate annealing temperature. If there is no access to a gradient PCR thermocycler, touchdown PCR can be applied to increase the annealing sensitivity.
2. PCR reaction system: A commercially available PCR Master-Mix which mixes *Taq* DNA polymerase and dNTP with optimal salt concentration can be easily used for bisulfite PCR. If this common PCR reaction system cannot produce a clean band, it is advisable to try a different PCR reaction system. In

our laboratory, we normally use FastStart Taq polymerase from Roche to improve the bisulfite PCR results (*see* **Note 3**).

PCR cycling conditions	
1. 94 °C	5 min
2. 95 °C	30 s
3. 55 °C	30 s
4. 72 °C	30 s
5. Go to 2	39 cycles
6. 74 °C	10 min
7. 4 °C	∞

PCR mix	
FMR1 F primer (2 μM)	1 μL
FMR1 R primer (2 μM)	1 μL
dNTPs (10 mM)	0.5 μL
FastSart Buffer containing $MgCl_2$	2.5 μL
FastStar taq	0.3 μL
Converted DNA	2 μL
DDW	12.7 μL

3. Visualized the PCR products by agarose gel electrophoresis and analyses by cloning and sequencing. Run 5 μL PCR products on 1.5% Agarose gel in order to verify the specificity of the primers. A single appropriately sized band indicates successful PCR amplification.

3.1.3 Bisulfite Colony Sequencing

1. *PCR purification products.* Commercially available kits such as the RBC Kit for specific PCR fragment purification and Gel Extraction can help to isolate the target PCR product from multiple nonspecific PCR bands.
2. *PCR cloning.* Clone sequencing is necessary to observe the distribution of methylation patterns at the single molecule level. For this purpose we use pGEM-T Easy vector system II (Promega) which provides the T4 DNA ligase system, a pGEM-T Easy vector and competent DH5α cells as well. By using this kit, purified PCR products can be ligated to the pGEM-T Easy vector and transformed into competent DH5α cells. The DH5α cells that carry the ligated vectors can be selected on agar plates containing ampicillin/X-gal/IPTG by

color change where blue colonies represent empty vector, and white colonies represent vectors inserted with target PCR products. The white colonies can then be selected and grown in LB medium + ampicillin. Plasmids containing target DNA are extracted by using a Miniprep Kit (RBC), then subjected to colony PCR and standard sequencing analysis.

3. *Colony PCR*. Mini prep products are subjected to a PCR reaction with SP6 and T7 primers.

Ready mix (×5)	5 μL
SP6 (2 μM)	1.5 μL
T7 (2 μM)	1.5 μL
Mini prep product	1 μL
DDW	16 μL

4. *Direct PCR Sequencing*. Single colonies are analyzed for CpG methylation by direct sequencing (ABI 3130). After cloning and sequencing, the methylation state of individual molecules can be tabulated, in a bisulfite map, to visualize the percent of methylation.

Sequencing reaction	
1. 96 °C	2 min
2. 96 °C	10s
3. 50 °C	5 s
4. 60 °C	4 min
5. Go to 2	25 times
6. 10 °C	∞

Sequencing mix	
BigDye 3.1 V	1.2 μL
BigDye Buffer	3.4 μL
Primer (10 μM) SP6/T7	0.8 μL
Colony PCR product	2-3 μL
DDW	11.6 μL

5. *Purify sequencing products.* Performa DTR (Dye Terminator Removal) Gel Filtration Cartridges are 800 μL spin columns assembled in a 1.5 mL microcentrifuge tube. These columns provide optimal performance for removal of unincorporated BigDye® v1.1, v3.0, and v3.1 and other dye terminators, dNTPs, salts, and other low molecular weight materials from sequencing reactions. These columns also remove DNA primers and fragments up to 20 bases, buffers, and nucleotides labeled with biotin, isotopes, and other assorted markers.
6. Centrifuge the Performa Gel Filtration Cartridge (BigDye® v3.1) for 3 min at 850 × *g*.
7. Remove the spin column and transfer to the provided 1.5 mL microcentrifuge tube.
8. Add the reaction sample of 10–20 μL to the center of each column.
9. Centrifuge for 3 min at 850 × *g*. Retain eluate.
   - Up to 4 μL may be lost during sample processing.
   - If the volume loss is greater than 4 μL, this is an indication of an overly dry gel. To optimize recovery of sample, repeat centrifugation.

3.1.4 Deep-Sequencing Analysis

16S Library Preparation and Deep-sequencing. A D1000 ScreenTape kit (Agilent Technologies) and Qubit® DNA HSAssay kit (Invitrogen) are used for quality control of PCR amplicons, followed by bead purification (×1, Agencourt AMPure XP—Beckman Coulter), according to the manufacturer's protocol. Subsequently, the amplicons are subjected to a second PrimMax Takara PCR reaction (first purified PCR DNA (7.5 μL), 2.5 μL N7XX primer (nextera barcode 1), 2.5 μL S5XX primer (nextera barcode 2), 12.5 μL 2× Primstar ReadyMix). The PCR program is: 98 °C for 1 min followed by 8 cycles of: 98 °C for 10 s, 55 °C for 10 s, 72 °C for 30 s, then 72 °C for 5 min and a hold at 10 °C. The second PCR is bead purified, followed by the use of the ScreenTape kit and the Qubit® DNA HS Assay kit for quality control and normalization of prepared libraries. Samples are pooled at 10 nM concentration, and then diluted to 4 nM for denaturation according to the Illumina protocol. A multiplexed sample pool (1.5 pM including PhiX 40%) is then loaded into the NextSeq 500 Mid-Output Kit (150 cycles) cartridge (Illumina, San Diego, CA) and loaded onto a NextSeq 500 System instrument (Illumina), with 150 cycles and single-read sequencing conditions. Data analysis: Raw sequence reads are mapped to the human genome (build GRCh38). Methylation calls are extracted after duplicate sequences had been excluded. Data visualization and analysis are performed using custom R and Java scripts. CpG methylation is calculated as the average of methylation for each CpG position, and non-CpG methylation is extracted from Bismark reports.

3.2 Monitoring for Histone Modifications at the FMR1 Locus by Chromatin Immunoprecipitation Assay

3.2.1 In Vivo Cross-Linking

1. Grow the cells until they reach ~80–90% confluence (attached cells) or in suspension. For human embryonic stem cells grow under feeder free conditions on vitronectin, with the E8 supplemented medium (Gibco) on 6-well dishes we use ~5-6 plates that are equivalent to approximately 2×10^7 cells. This will provide a chromatin preparation that can be used for up to 10 separate immunoprecipitation reactions.
2. De-attach the cells with trypsin–EDTA, 0.5 mL per well during 5 min at 37 °C.
3. Neutralize the trypsin by addition of full hESC growth medium containing serum.
4. Collect the cells into a 50 mL tube, spin down the cells (5 min, 10,000 × *g*) and discard supernatant.
5. Wash the cells with PBSX1, spin down the cells (5 min, 10,000 × *g*) and remove supernatant.
6. Resuspend the cells into 10 mL full medium. Count the cells and fix the concentration to $2–2.2 \times 10^6$ cell per mL with full hESC growth medium.
7. Add 270 μL of 37% formaldehyde to 10 mL of growth media to cross-link while gently swirling the tube (*see* **Note 4**). Final concentration of the formaldehyde is 1%. Use high quality formaldehyde. Do not use if formaldehyde is past expiration date as suggested by the manufacturer.
8. Incubate at room temperature for 10 min.
9. Add 1 mL of 1.25 M Glycine to the tube to quench unreacted formaldehyde. Swirl to mix and incubate at room temperature for 5 min.
10. Centrifuge for 3 min at 700 × *g* at 4 °C.
11. Aspirate the medium by removing as much medium as possible and add 10 mL cold PBSX1.
12. Centrifuge for 3 min at 700 × *g* at 4 °C.
13. Remove the PBS and repeat PBS washes step.
14. Add 1 mL cold PBSX1 containing 2.5 μL Protease inhibitor cocktail II(X400) and transfer the cells to eppendorf tube.
15. Spin at 700 × *g* at 4 °C for 5 min to pellet the cells.
16. Discard supernatant.
17. Flash-freeze the cells in liquid nitrogen and store in −80 °C or continue to the chromatin purification step.

3.2.2 Lysis and Chromatin Purification

1. Thaw the fixed cells pellets on ice.
2. Resuspend the cells with 1 mL SDS lysis buffer containing Protease Inhibitors cocktail II (*see* **Note 5**).
3. Incubate for 0.5–1 h on ice.
4. Aliquot 500 μL per microfuge tube, the cell lysate can be frozen at −80 °C at this step or continue to the sonication step.

3.2.3 DNA Shear by Bioruptor Sonication

1. If cell lysate was previously frozen, thaw on ice. Prepare: 1.5 mL tube containing the cells with the lysis buffer on fresh ice +1.5 mL tube for equilibration + a big beaker for excess water + timer + cold water. Set the small centrifuge to 4 °C.
2. Take out the water from the sonicator. Add the cold water to the sonicator 1 cm under the line. Add ice until the water reaches the line. Insert the 1.5 mL tubes to the sonicator and close lid. Make sure that it is set for high, 0.5 min on-0.5 min off.
3. Start the sonication for 7 min × 2 (the time of sonication should be optimized to reach a smear in the gel agarose with a peak at 200–300 bp following electrophoresis) (*see* **Note 6**).
4. Centrifuge the sheered chromatin for 15 min 4 °C, 10,000 × *g*.
5. Divide the supernatant into the ChIP vials, 100 μL each containing 2.2×10^6 cell equivalents which is enough for one immunoprecipitation.
6. You can stop at this stage and store the samples at −80 °C after freezing with liquid nitrogen. Sheared cross-linked chromatin can be stored at −80 °C for up to a few months.

3.2.4 Validation of Sonication

1. Dilute the Input (use half of the Input) samples with up to 100 μL with Elution buffer and add 5 M NaCl to a final concentration of 0.2 M NaCl.
2. Add RNase (DNase free) and incubate for 30 min, 37 °C, shaking at 10,000 × *g*.
3. Add Proteinase K and reverse cross-link for 3 h, at 65 °C, shaking at 10,000 × *g*.
4. Purify using PCR/gel extraction kit and run the sonicated samples on a gel to obtain a smear which should have a peak at ~300 bp. Run 1–1.5 μg of the input in a 1.5% agarose gel, 80 V for 30 min.

3.2.5 Immunoprecipitation (IP) First Day

1. Thaw the chromatin slowly; keep it cold at all times. Remove from −20 °C the Protease Inhibitor Cocktail II (PI II) and thaw at room temperature.
2. Prepare enough Dilution Buffer containing protease inhibitors for the number of desired immunoprecipitations and store on

ice. Each IP requires the addition of 900 μL of Dilution Buffer and 4.5 μL of Protease Inhibitor Cocktail II.

3. Add 900 μL of Dilution Buffer containing PIC II into each tube containing 100 μL of chromatin.
4. Remove 10 μL of the supernatant as "Input" and save at 4 °C.
5. Add the immunoprecipitating antibody and 30 μL fully suspended protein G magnetic beads (*see* **Note** 7).
6. Incubate overnight at 4 °C with rotation 12 h (do not exceed 14 h).

3.2.6 Immunoprecipitation (IP) Second Day

1. Pellet protein G magnetic beads with the magnetic separator and remove the supernatant completely.
2. Wash the protein G bead-antibody–chromatin complex by resuspending the beads in 1 mL each of the cold buffers in the order listed below (all the buffers can be stored up to 1 year at 4 °C) and incubating for 3–5 min on a rotating platform followed by magnetic clearance and careful removal of the supernatant fraction:
   (a) Low Salt Immune Complex Wash Buffer, one wash.
   (b) High Salt Immune Complex Wash Buffer, one wash.
   (c) LiCl Immune Complex Wash Buffer, one wash.
   (d) TE Buffer, one wash.

3.2.7 Elution of Protein–DNA Complexes and Reverse Cross-Links of Protein–DNA Complexes to Free DNA

1. Thaw Proteinase K and warm the ChIP Elution Buffer to room temperature.
2. Add 300 μL Elution Buffer to the beads and to the input.
3. Add 1 μL RNaseA and incubate for 30 min at 37 °C, 600 rpm shaking. Add 2 μL of 20 mg/mL Proteinase K and reverse histone–DNA cross-links by heating at 65 °C for 5 h-O/N.
4. Transfer the tubes to magnetic rack and collect the supernatant to new eppendorf.
5. Use PCR purification kit (RBC). Elute with 50 μL preheated elution buffer to 60 °C and then another 50 μL (total of 100 μL).

3.2.8 Detection

This is the most variable step of the procedure because of the number of detection methods that can be employed and the variability of PCR primer selection. The most meaningful results will be obtained with quantitative PCR for this step and Real Time Quantitative PCR (RT-qPCR) is ideal for implementation. Success in obtaining high-quality quantitative data is critically dependent on good primer design. In general, primers should be 20 to 30 bases long with a *Tm* of 55° to 60 °C and optimum GC content of 50%. Amplification products should be 100 to 300 bp. Longer PCR products should be avoided, because the amplification efficiency is substantially lower, and DNA fragments that do not bind to both primers will not be amplified (this can be a significant problem since the size of DNA fragments in the samples averages ~500 bp and ranges between 100 to 1000 bp). A final primer concentration of 0.5 μM works well for most primers, but in some instances, improved product specificity may be obtained by lowering the final primer concentration five- to tenfold.

Immunoprecipitated chromatin is analyzed using real-time PCR, looking for enrichments at the FMR1 promoter region, 300 bp upstream to the transcription start site (TSS). HoxA9 and APRT are used as positive and negative controls, respectively, for both H3K9me3 and H3K27me3; and APRT and Crystalin are used as positive and negative controls for H3K4me2, respectively. Enrichments (ΔΔCt) are normalized to positive controls, and FMR1 and negative controls are presented in graphs. The results can be presented also as relative enrichment with respect to the negative control. The positive control shows that the immunoprecipitation succeeded and the negative control gives the baseline noise of the assay. The data represents average values of three to five independent ChIP experiments. Error bars represent standard error (paired t test, $*p < 0.05$, $**p < 0.01$, $***p < 0.001$) (*see* **Note 8**).

$\Delta\Delta C_t$ Calculation

$$\textbf{Average}\ C_t^{(\mathrm{INPUT})}\text{\_Average}\ C_t^{(\mathrm{IP})} = \Delta C_t$$

Subtract ΔC_t for the experimental primer pair from ΔC_t of the negative control $\Delta C_t^{\exp} - \Delta C_t^{\mathrm{control}} = \Delta\Delta C_t$

4 Notes

1. *Completeness of bisulfite conversion*

   After bisulfite conversion PCR analysis is often the first indicator to evaluate the success of the bisulfite conversion. For a pilot experiment, select gDNA of known purity and quantity, not exceeding 300 ng for a 150 μL bisulfite conversion reaction. The most common sources of poor bisulfite conversion are from insufficient denaturation due to excess gDNA concentration or poor sample purity and possible renaturation of the freshly denatured gDNA. Testing XX normal cells for FMR1 methylation can serve as a 50/50 methylated/nonmethylated control for bisulfite conversion efficiency.

2. *Primer design*

   Primers designed outside of a CpG region of interest will, in principle, amplify the target regardless of the methylation state

of the internal sequence. Bisulfite sequencing provides an inherently more accurate assessment of the methylation state of a sample compared to PCR primers (or probes) that select for presupposed fully methylated or fully unmethylated complementary sequences, such as Methyl specific primers.
Methyl Primer Express® Software is a free online primer design tool (geared specifically to facilitate methylation studies) which assists primer design for both methylated and unmethylated bisulfite modified DNA. Users simply cut and paste in the selected genomic sequence, the software then performs an in silico bisulfite conversion (C's are converted to T's), and aids in the selection of primers. Methyl Primer Express software is available for free downloads at: (http://marketing.appliedbiosystems.com/mk/get/GAAS_CLINICAL_METHYLATED?_A=77005&_D=50613&_V=0#).

3. *PCR bias which is a variable for each sample and each analysis*

   Bisulfite PCR amplification can be performed as a regular PCR reaction. However, PCR conditions for amplifying bisulfite-treated material should be carefully optimized since the bisulfite treatment reduces the specificity of DNA double strands. It is recommended to use 1–4 μL of eluted DNA for each PCR, however, up to 10 μL can be used if necessary. The elution volume can be ≥10 μL depending on the requirements of the experiment but small elution volumes will yield more concentrated DNA.

4. *Cross-linking*

   This treatment cross-links the proteins to the DNA ensuring coprecipitation of the DNA with the protein of interest.
   The extent of formaldehyde cross-linking is an important variable that in principle may be modified by changing the duration of cross-linking, the concentration of formaldehyde, or the temperature at which the cross-linking is performed. For some applications where protein cross-linking is particularly efficient (as for histones) it might be useful to decrease the cross-linking time or formaldehyde concentration. In particular, histone tails have a number of lysine residues that are likely to be modified by formaldehyde, and such modified lysine may interfere with the binding of antibodies against specific peptides corresponding to modified histones (e.g., by acetylation, phosphorylation, methylation).

5. *Cell lysis*

   Although complete lysis of all cells is not absolutely necessary (and may be difficult to achieve), it is very important that lysis be as efficient as possible. Efficient lysis is important to obtain a reproducible degree of cell breakage among a group of samples to reliably compare results. Significant differences in cell lysis efficiency will result in immunoprecipitations with different ratios of antibody to chromatin, which will possibly alter immunoprecipitation efficiency.

6. *Sonication*

Shearing DNA to a small size (~500 bp average) by sonication is the critical factor in achieving resolution between a DNA sequence where a particular protein is bound and a nearby (*cis*-) DNA sequence that does not bind that protein. In addition, fragmentation of the chromatin is essential for its solubilization from the ruptured cells. The ability to fragment and solubilize the chromatin depends on the extent of chromatin cross-linking. In general, more cross-linking results in larger fragment size and lower solubility, resulting in lower yield. Because of the importance of this variable, the DNA size should be assessed to confirm that the desired degree of fragmentation has been achieved, and it should be reassessed if fixation conditions are change.

Optimization of DNA Sonication.

Optimal conditions required for shearing cross-linked DNA to 200–1000 base pairs in length depend on the cell type, cell concentration per lysis buffer and the sonicator equipment, including the power settings and number of pulses. Following the protocol below, determine the optimal conditions required.

(a) Generate at least four different microfuge tubes containing a variety of cell equivalent concentrations in the range of 5×10^6 per mL to 5×10^7 per mL. Each microfuge tube should contain approximately 300–400 μL of cell lysate.

(b) Be sure to keep the samples on ice at all times during the sonication processes, as sonication generates heat which will denature the chromatin.

(c) Remove 1×10^5 cell equivalents from each condition prior to sonication for analysis of unsheared DNA.

(d) For each cell concentration, sonicate each tube for a different number of 10 s pulses depending on the number of tubes. For example, sonicate the first tube for 1×10 s, the second tube for 2×10 s, the third tube for 3×10 s and the fourth tube for 4×10 s.

(e) Repeat for all cell concentrations.

(f) Remove 5 μL of the sonicated chromatin from each condition to a fresh tube.

(g) To all 5 μL samples (unsheared and sheared), add 90 μL ddH_2O and 4 μL 5 M NaCl.

(h) Incubate for at least 4–5 h to overnight at 65 °C to reverse the DNA–protein cross-links.

(i) Add 1 μL of RNase A and incubate for 30 min at 37 °C.

(j) Add 2 μL 0.5 M EDTA, 4 μL 1 M Tris–HCl and 1 μL Proteinase K and incubate at 45 °C for 1–2 h.

(k) Load 10 μL (1×10^4 cell equivalents) and 20 μL (2×10^4 cell equivalents) on a 1–2% agarose gel with a 100 bp DNA marker.

- Loading different amounts helps to avoid underloading or overloading.

(l) Observe which of the shearing conditions gives a smear of DNA in the range of 200 bp–1000 bp.

(m) Repeat optimization of the shearing conditions if the results indicate that the fragmented DNA is not in the desired size range. Once optimal conditions have been determined, it is advised that the user does not alter the cell concentration or volume of lysate per microfuge tube for subsequent chromatin immunoprecipitation experiments.

7. *Immunoprecipitation*

The success of this procedure relies on the use of an antibody that will specifically and tightly bind its target protein in the buffer and wash conditions used. In addition, the antibody should be present in excess with respect to its target protein so that differences in the amount of protein–DNA complexes of interest will be accurately measured. When quantitative PCR will be performed in real time using SYBR Green, high-quality primer pairs should result in ~1.9-fold amplification/cycle. Such amplification efficiency can be determined from quantitative analysis of raw fluorescence data for each cycle. Amplification efficiencies <1.8 are likely to cause problems, particularly if detection of the PCR product requires 30 cycles or more. Specificity information may also be obtained by running dissociation curves on reactions following the conclusion of the PCR run.

8. *Quantitation*

When quantitative PCR is performed in real time using SYBR Green, the linear range is directly visualized and the quality of the reactions can be directly assessed. For reactions involving a given primer, the curves should be superimposable with respect to shape, and they should differ only in the number of cycles needed to reach the threshold (*Ct*). Amplification efficiencies should be ~1.9-fold/cycle. If the curves have different shapes and/or amplification efficiencies are <1.8, the reactions are not equivalent and accurate quantitation is impossible.

(a) *Controls*

The control, which is usually meaningful, is to examine a given pair of input and immunoprecipitated samples for multiple genomic regions. Control genomic regions should all give the same background level of apparent immunoprecipitation efficiency. Fragments bound by the protein of interest will give higher apparent immunoprecipitation efficiencies, and the difference can be expressed as fold enrichment over the background level. In the best cases, enrichments can be >100-fold, but even a factor of two can be meaningful if the experiment is repeated enough times and the experimentally determined error is sufficiently low. The advantage of this approach is that identical samples are used to directly determine relative protein association to different genomic regions. Furthermore, differences in fold enrichment for different genomic regions represent relative quantitative measurements of protein association in vivo.

(b) *Data interpretation*

In most experiments, it is presumed that the protein of interest associates specifically with certain genomic regions and associates only nonspecifically with other genomic regions. In general, it is very difficult to distinguish true nonspecific association from experimental background of the cross-linking procedure. In this regard, immunoprecipitations with the antibody of interest generally give two- to threefold higher immunoprecipitation efficiencies than immunoprecipitations with control (or no) antibodies, but it is unclear whether this effect is physiologically meaningful or an experimental artifact. Moreover, for a given pair of INPUT and IP samples, the fold enrichment of a given genomic region over the background is directly related to the level of protein association in vivo. It is useful to define "relative protein occupancies" for different regions by subtracting the background from the observed immunoprecipitation efficiencies. For some experiments, particularly those involving histone modifications, it is inappropriate to analyze the data in terms of occupancy units and specific versus nonspecific binding sites. Histones associate with essentially all genomic regions, and the level of a particular chromatin modification typically occurs in a continuum. Thus, it is very difficult to determine whether a given region is devoid of a particular modification, although information in this regard can be obtained in control immunoprecipitations using an off-target antibody. For these reasons, quantitative analysis of the relative level of a given histone modification is best presented using simple immunoprecipitation efficiencies. Again, to account for sample-to-sample variations, a specific genomic region should be given an arbitrarily defined value, which is used to determine the relative levels of all other genomic regions.

References

1. Verkerk AJ, Pieretti M, Sutcliffe JS, Fu YH, Kuhl DP, Pizzuti A et al (1991) Identification of a gene (FMR-1) containing a CGG repeat coincident with a breakpoint cluster region exhibiting length variation in fragile X syndrome. Cell 65:905–914. https://doi.org/10.1016/0092-8674(91)90397-h
2. Oberlé I, Rousseau F, Heitz D, Kretz C, Devys D, Hanauer A et al (1991) Instability of a 550-base pair DNA segment and abnormal methylation in fragile X syndrome. Science 252:1097–1102. https://doi.org/10.1126/science.252
3. Hayward BE, Kumari D, Usdin K (2017) Recent advances in assays for the fragile X-related disorders. Hum Genet 136(10):1313–1327. Review
4. Coffee B, Zhang F, Ceman S, Warren ST, Reines D (2002) Histone modifications depict an aberrantly heterochromatinized FMR1 gene in fragile x syndrome. Am J Hum Genet 71:923–932
5. Coffee B, Zhang F, Warren ST, Reines D (1999) Acetylated histones are associated with FMR1 in normal but not fragile X-syndrome cells. Nat Genet 22:98–101
6. Pietrobono R, Tabolacci E, Zalfa F, Zito I, Terracciano A, Moscato U (2005) Molecular dissection of the events leading to inactivation of the FMR1 gene. Hum Mol Genet 14:267–277
7. Tabolacci E, Moscato U, Zalfa F, Bagni C, Chiurazzi P, Neri G (2008) Epigenetic analysis reveals a euchromatic configuration in the FMR1 unmethylated full mutations. Eur J Hum Genet 16:1487–1498
8. Tabolacci E, Pietrobono R, Moscato U, Oostra BA, Chiurazzi P, Neri G (2005) Differential epigenetic modifications in the FMR1 gene of the fragile X syndrome after reactivating pharmacological treatments. Eur J Hum Genet 13:641–648
9. Kumari D, Usdin K (2010) The distribution of repressive histone modifications on silenced FMR1 alleles provides clues to the mechanism of gene silencing in fragile X syndrome. Hum Mol Genet 19(23):4634–4642

Chapter 4

Assays for Determining Repeat Number, Methylation Status, and AGG Interruptions in the Fragile X-Related Disorders

Bruce E. Hayward and Karen Usdin

Abstract

Knowledge of the CGG•CCG-repeat number, AGG interruption status, and the extent of DNA methylation of the *FMR1* gene are vital for both diagnosis of the fragile X-related disorders and for basic research into disease mechanisms. We describe here assays that we use in our laboratory to assess these parameters. Our assays are PCR-based and include one for repeat size that can also be used to assess the extent of methylation and a related assay that allows the AGG interruption pattern to be reliably determined even in women. A second more quantitative methylation assay is also described. We also describe our method for cloning of repeats to generate the reference standards necessary for the accurate determination of repeat number and AGG interruption status.

Key words *FMR1*-related disorders (*FMR1* disorders), FX-associated tremor and ataxia syndrome (FXTAS), FX-associated primary ovarian insufficiency (FXPOI), Fragile X syndrome (FXS), Repeat PCR, AGG PCR assay, Quantitative methylation assay, *FMR1*, qPCR, AGG interruptions

1 Introduction

The mutation responsible for the fragile X-related disorders is an expansion of a CGG•CCG-repeat tract in exon 1 of the X-linked gene, *FMR1* [1]. As discussed elsewhere in this volume, the symptoms of these disorders are related to the repeat number, with alleles having 55–200 repeats conferring risk of fragile X-associated tremor/ataxia and fragile X-associated primary ovarian insufficiency and alleles with >200 repeats resulting in fragile X syndrome. However, the repeat tract is difficult to amplify by PCR likely because of the secondary structures formed by the repeats [2]. This difficulty is compounded by the mosaicism that is often present in affected individuals [3]. The risk of further expansion on maternal transmission is related to both the repeat number and the number of AGG interruptions. Thus, it is important to be able to

Grant Sponsor: Intramural program of the NIDDK, NIH (DK057808)

Dalit Ben-Yosef and Yoav Mayshar (eds.), *Fragile-X Syndrome: Methods and Protocols*, Methods in Molecular Biology, vol. 1942, https://doi.org/10.1007/978-1-4939-9080-1_4, © Springer Science+Business Media, LLC, part of Springer Nature 2019

reliably determine this second parameter, particularly in females [4–7]. However, the presence of a second X chromosome can make doing so quite challenging. Finally, expansion beyond 200 repeats results in repeat-mediated gene silencing, the extent of which affects symptom severity. Methylation mosaicism is also present in many individuals [3]. Thus, quantitative assays for DNA methylation are also an important tool in the diagnostic toolbox. The ability to accurately measure repeat number and methylation status is also important in a research setting since the cell lines that are frequently used can sometimes show both variations in repeat number and the extent of DNA methylation [8, 9]. We describe here the PCR methods that we use in our laboratory to determine all the parameters necessary for a complete genetic workup or thorough laboratory study, including an assay that can be used to unambiguously ascertain the number of AGG interruptions even in women and a quantitative assay for the methylation status that is useful even in the case of extensive methylation mosaicism. We also describe how to generate suitable standards for the accurate determination of both the repeat number and the AGG interruption status.

2 Materials

2.1 Repeat PCR Assay

1. 10× PCR buffer: 500 mM Tris–HCl pH 9.0, 15 mM $MgCl_2$, 220 mM $(NH_4)_2SO_4$ (*see* **Note 1**), 2% Triton X-100. Store at room temperature.
2. 5 M betaine: Weigh 33.8 g betaine monohydrate and add water to give a final volume of 50 ml. Filter through a 0.2 μm filter to sterilize. Store at 4 °C.
3. DMSO. Store at room temperature in the dark.
4. dNTP solution: 10 mM each (*see* **Note 2**),
5. Primers:
   - (a) Not_FraxC (5′-**AGTTCAGCGGCCGC**GCTCAGCTCCGTTTCGGTTTCACTTCCGGT-3′),
   - (b) Not_FraxR4 (5′-**CAAGTCGCGGCCGC**CTTGTAGAAAGCGCCATTGGAGCCCCGCA-3′).

   Prepare working stocks of 10 μm of each primer in water (*see* **Note 3**). For fragment analysis by capillary electrophoresis Not_FraxR4 should be labeled with a fluorophore.
6. Thermostable polymerase: Q5® Hot Start polymerase (New England Biolabs; *see* **Note 4**).
7. Restriction enzymes: HindIII and HpaII. Store at −20 °C (*see* **Note 5**).

8. Genomic DNA: High molecular weight DNA prepared from cells by the salting out method [10] or from saliva using Oragene reagents (DNA Genotek; *see* **Note 6**).
9. CGG-repeat size markers for capillary electrophoresis (*see* **Note 7**).

2.2 AGG PCR Assays

1. 10× AGG PCR buffer: 500 mM Tris–HCl pH 9.0, 17.5 mM $MgCl_2$, 220 mM $(NH_4)_2SO_4$ (*see* **Note 1**). Store at room temperature.
2. 5 M betaine: Weigh 33.8 g betaine monohydrate and add water to give a final volume of 50 ml. Filter through a 0.2 μm filter to sterilize. Store at 4 °C.
3. DMSO. Store at room temperature in the dark.
4. dNTP solution: 10 mM each (*see* **Note 2**),
5. Primers:
   (a) Not_FraxC (5′-FAM-**AGTTCAGCGGCCGC**GCTCAGCTCCGTTTCGGTTTCACTTCCGGT-3′),
   (b) Not_FraxR4 (5′-HEX-**CAAGTCGCGGCCGC**CTTGTAGAAAGCGCCATTGGAGCCCCGCA-3′),
   (c) Not_PsdR4 (5′-NED-**CAAGTCGCGGCCGC**AGCCGCGAGAAATGCCTCCTGCGCAATGT-3′),
   (d) A-primer (5′-**AGCGTCTACTGTCTCGGCACTGT**CGGCGGCGGA-3′),
   (e) T-primer (5′-**AGCGTCTACTGTCTCGGCACTTGC**CCGCCGCCGCCT-3′).

   Prepare working stocks of 10 μM of each primer in water (*see* **Note 3**). If Not_PsdR4 is to be incorporated into the reaction as a positive control, make a combined working stock with Not_FraxR4 with both at 10 μM each.
6. Thermostable polymerase: KAPA2G Robust Hot Start (KAPA Biosystems; *see* **Note 8**).
7. Restriction enzyme: HindIII. Store at −20 °C (*see* **Note 5**).
8. Genomic DNA: High molecular weight DNA prepared from cells by the salting out method [10] or from saliva using Oragene reagents (*see* **Note 6**).
9. CGG-repeat size markers carrying known AGG interruption patterns (*see* **Note 7**).

2.3 Quantitative Methylation Assay

1. Restriction enzyme: HpaII. Store at −20 °C.
2. Genomic DNA: High molecular weight DNA prepared from cells by the salting out method [10] or from saliva using Oragene reagents (*see* **Note 6**).

3. Primers:
   (a) FMR1 ex1 F (5′-GAACAGCGTTGATCACGTGAC-3′).
   (b) FMR1 ex1 R (5′-GTGAAACCGAAACGGAGCTGA-3′).
   (c) GAPDH ex1 F (5′-TCGACAGTCAGCCGCATCT-3′).
   (d) GAPDH int1 R (5′-CTAGCCTCCCGGGTTTCTCT-3′). Prepare working stocks of 10 μm of each primer in water (*see* **Note 3**).
4. Power SYBR Green Master Mix (ThermoFisher Scientific)

2.4 Generation of Reference Standards

1. 10× PCR buffer: 500 mM Tris–HCl pH 9.0, 15 mM $MgCl_2$, 220 mM $(NH_4)_2SO_4$ (*see* **Note 1**), 2% Triton X-100. Store at room temperature.
2. 5 M betaine: Weigh 33.8 g betaine monohydrate and add water to give a final volume of 50 ml. Filter through a 0.2 μM filter to sterilize. Store at 4 °C.
3. DMSO. Store at room temperature in the dark.
4. dNTP solution: 10 mM each (*see* **Note 2**),
5. Primers:
   (a) Gb_FraxC (5′-**CTGGAGCAATTCCGGCGCGCCG**CTCAGCTCCGTTTCGGTTTCACTTCCGGT-3′),
   (b) Gb_FraxR4 (5′-**CTCGCCCTTGCTCACCATGG**GAACATCCTTTACAAATGCCTTGTAGAAAGCGCCATTGGAGCCCCGCA-3′).
   (c) 612F (5′- ATAAGCTTTAGGCGTGTACGG-3′).
   (d) 1311R (5′- CGCTGAACTTGTGGCCGTTTA-3′).

   Prepare working stocks of 10 μM of each primer in water (*see* **Note 3**).
6. Thermostable polymerase: Q5® Hot Start (New England Biolabs).
7. Restriction enzymes: HindIII. Store at −20 °C (*see* **Note 5**).
8. Genomic DNA: High molecular weight DNA prepared from cells by the salting out method [10] or from saliva using Oragene reagents (*see* **Note 6**).
9. Addgene plasmid 99255 (*see* **Note 7**).

3 Methods

3.1 Restriction Enzyme Digestion of Genomic DNA

This protocol is required for both the Repeat PCR and AGG PCR assays.

1. Assemble a 40 μl reaction containing 4 μl of the appropriate 10× PCR buffer (either Repeat PCR buffer or AGG PCR buffer), 600 ng of genomic DNA (*see* **Note 6**), and 1 μl of

HindIII restriction enzyme (20 U in the case of HindIII-HF from New England Biolabs). Mix well.

2. If the methylation status of the alleles is to be tested (only applicable to the Repeat assay PCR), divide the reaction into 2 × 20 μl aliquots and add 0.5 μl of HpaII (5 U in the case of HpaII from New England Biolabs) to one aliquot. Mix well.
3. Incubate overnight at 37 °C in either a heating block with a heated lid set at 45 °C or in a 37 °C air incubator to reduce evaporation (*see* **Note 9**).

3.2 Repeat PCR Assay

1. Assemble the PCR master mix to give sufficient volume for N + 1 PCR reactions (*see* **Note 10**). The following volumes are for 10 PCR reactions (i.e., 9 + 1): 15 μl 10× PCR buffer, 10 μl 10 μM Not_FraxC, 10 μl 10 μM Not_FraxR4, 100 μl 5 M betaine, 4 μl DMSO, 9 μl dNTP solution (*see* **Note 11**), and 2 μl Q5® polymerase. Mixing the betaine and 10× PCR buffer together turns the solution cloudy momentarily.
2. Place 5 μl of the digestion reactions into a PCR tube and then add 15 μl of the PCR master mix, pipetting gently up and down several times to ensure that the solutions are completely mixed.
3. Initiate the PCR program and wait until the block has reached at least 70 °C before putting the tubes in. Cycle for: 98 °C 3 min, 30 × (98 °C 30 s, 59 °C 30 s, 72 °C 210 s), 72 °C 10 min, then hold at 12 °C or store at −20 °C until ready to analyze.
4. The products can be analyzed by agarose gel electrophoresis. However, ethidium bromide has been reported to alter the mobility of CGG-repeat containing fragments [11], so the gel should be run without ethidium bromide and stained afterward. An approximate repeat number can be calculated as follows: (fragment size-270)/3.
5. For more accurate size determinations, the samples can be analyzed by capillary electrophoresis if one of the primers used was fluorescently labeled (*see* **Note 7**).

3.3 AGG PCR Assays

1. The A-primed assay is used to determine the number of AGG interruptions in each allele. The T-primed assay can be used subsequently for a more accurate determination of the interspersion pattern if needed (see [13] for a more detailed discussion). Assemble the PCR master mix to give sufficient volume for N + 1 PCR reactions (*see* **Note 10**). The following volumes are for 10 A-primed PCR reactions without the positive control (i.e., 9 + 1): 15 μl 10× AGG PCR buffer, 10 μl 10 μM A-primer, 10 μl 10 μM HEX-labeled Not_FraxR4, 100 μl 5 M betaine, 4 μl DMSO, 4 μl dNTP solution, 5.5 μl H_2O, and 1.5 μl KAPA2G polymerase. For 10 A-primed PCR

reactions with the positive control: 15 μl 10× AGG PCR buffer, 10 μl 10 μM A-primer, 10 μl (10 μM HEX-labeled Not_FraxR4 + 10 μM NED-labeled Not_PsdR4), 100 μl 5 M betaine, 4 μl DMSO, 4 μl dNTP solution, 1 μl 1 pg/ μl Addgene plasmid 99257 (*see* **Note 12**), 4.5 μl H_2O, and 1.5 μl KAPA2G polymerase. For 10 T-primed PCR reactions: 15 μl 10× AGG PCR buffer, 10 μl 10 μM T-primer, 10 μl 10 μM FAM-labeled Not_FraxC, 100 μl 5 M betaine, 4 μl DMSO, 4 μl dNTP solution, 5.5 μl H_2O, and 1.5 μl KAPA2G polymerase.

2. Place 5 μl of the digestion reactions into a PCR tube and then add 15 μl of the PCR master mix, pipetting gently up and down several times to ensure that the solutions are completely mixed (*see* **Note 10**).
3. Initiate the PCR program and wait until the block has reached at least 70 °C before putting the tubes in. Cycle for: 98 °C 3 min, 30 × (98 °C 30 s, 55 °C 30 s, 72 °C 210 s), 72 °C 10 min, then hold at 12 °C or store at −20 °C until ready to visualize.
4. Agarose gel electrophoresis is not suitable for the analysis of these reaction products due to priming by the A-primer/T-primer elsewhere in the genome. Thus, capillary electrophoresis with the appropriate reference standards must be used (*see* **Note 7**). Note that if the positive control plasmid for the A-primed assay is incorporated as indicated above there will be a NED-labeled fragment present in the "water-only" PCR control.

3.4 Quantitative Methylation Assay

1. Make a 100 μl volume of genomic DNA at 10 ng/μl in H_2O.
2. Sonicate to fragment the DNA to 0.5–1 kb in size. This can be done using a Bioruptor (Diagenode) set at medium with cycles of 30 s on and 30 s off for 5 min (*see* **Note 13**). Verify the size by agarose gel electrophoresis of ~100 ng of the sample (*see* **Note 14**).
3. Combine 60 μl sonicated DNA (600 ng) with 10 μl 10 × CutSmart® buffer (New England Biolabs) and 25 μl H_2O.
4. Take two 45 μl aliquots and add 5 μl H_2O to one (mock digest) and 1.2 μl HpaII (*see* **Note 14**) + 3.8 μl H_2O to the other (to give 12 U HpaII digesting 300 ng DNA). Incubate overnight at 37 °C in either a heating block with a heated lid set at 45 °C or in a 37 °C air incubator to minimize evaporation-related problems. Heat-inactivate the HpaII by incubating at 80 °C for 20 min.
5. Each DNA sample requires 10 PCR replicates for the *FMR1* methylation assay (five undigested and five digested) and 6 PCR replicates for the *GAPDH* digestion control assay (three undigested and three digested). A master mix of ten

PCR reactions contains 100 µl Power SYBR Green Mix (2×), 4 µl 10 µM forward primer, 4 µl 10 µM reverse primer and 72 µl H_2O. For the *FMR1* methylation assay the primers are FMR1 ex1 F and FMR1 ex1 R while for the *GAPDH* digestion control the primers are GAPDH ex1 F and GAPDH int1 R. Make sufficient Master Mix to accommodate (No. of samples × No. of replicates) + 1.

6. Aliquot 10 × 18 µl of the *FMR1* methylation Master Mix into 10 wells of a qPCR 96-well plate and add 5 × 2 µl of the undigested DNA and 5 × 2 µl of the digested DNA. Similarly, aliquot 6 × 18 µl of the *GAPDH* digestion control Master Mix and add 3 × 2 µl of the undigested DNA and 3 × 2 µl of the digested DNA. Repeat for the remainder of the DNA samples.
7. Seal the 96-well plate. Centrifuge at 215 × *g* for 1 min.
8. Perform the qPCR using the following cycling parameters: 95 °C 10 min, 40 × (95 °C 15 s, 60 °C 60 s). Analyze the data by setting the Ct threshold to 0.1. Calculate the extent of digestion by taking the average of the Ct values of the undigested *GAPDH* qPCRs and the average of the Ct values of the digested *GAPDH* qPCRs and calculating the ΔCt value ($Ct_{digested} - Ct_{undigested}$). Digestion is complete if the value of $1/(2^{\Delta Ct})$ is ≤0.1.
   Calculate the *FMR1* methylation percentage similarly: ΔCt = (Average $Ct_{digested}$ − average $Ct_{undigested}$). % methylation = $1/(2^{\Delta Ct})$.

3.5 Generation of Reference Standards

3.5.1 Cloning of Repeat Sequences for Use as Reference Standards

1. To generate the plasmid backbone use plasmid DNA from Addgene plasmid 99255 and digest 5–10 µg with AscI + NcoI to separate the 4.4 kb plasmid backbone from the 350 bp *FMR1* insert. Use agarose gel electrophoresis to separate the two fragments and gel purify the backbone fragment (*see* **Note 15**).
2. Digest genomic DNA with HindIII as detailed in Subheading 3.1 (*see* **Note 16**).
3. Perform a preparative scale Repeat PCR by combining 25 µl of the digested genomic DNA with 75 µl of the Repeat PCR master mix (*see* Subheadings 3.2, **steps 1** and **2**) containing Q5® polymerase. Divide into 5 × 20 µl aliquots.
4. Initiate the PCR program and place the PCR reactions in the block when it has reached ≥70 °C. Cycle for 98 °C 3 min, 23 × (98 °C 30 s, 59 °C 30 s, 72 °C 120 s), 72 °C 10 min. (*see* **Note 17**).
5. Purify the PCR product using a standard PCR column cleanup kit (e.g., Qiagen QiaQuick or NEB Monarch) and elute in the minimum volume of elution buffer. The fragment will be barely visible on an agarose gel.

6. Use a Gibson Assembly kit (e.g., New England Biolabs or Synthetic Genomics) and a ratio of ~5:1 PCR fragment–plasmid backbone to carry out a Gibson assembly according to the manufacturer's instructions. Electroporate into an *E. coli* strain suitable for the maintenance of repetitive sequences (e.g., Endura™ (Lucigen) or NEB® Stable (New England Biolabs)).
7. Choose at least ten colonies and grow 3 ml cultures overnight. Take an aliquot from each culture and make a glycerol stock and then use the remainder to prepare plasmid. Digest the plasmids with AscI + NcoI to identify those containing a correctly sized insert.
8. Verify the clones by sequencing them using primers 612F and 1311R.
9. Generate large quantities of plasmid DNA by inoculating 4 × 100 ml cultures directly from the glycerol stock and harvest while the culture is still in log phase (<10 h growth at 37 °C). Isolate the plasmid and purify the AscI + NcoI fragment containing the *FMR1* sequence by agarose gel electrophoresis.

3.5.2 Use of Reference Standards

1. The individual plasmids containing defined repeat numbers or genomic DNA templates of known repeat number and/or interspersion patterns should be amplified using the Repeat PCR protocol for the CGG size ladder or the AGG PCR protocol for the AGG interruption ladder using the same labeled primer as the samples to be analyzed.
2. After purification with a PCR column cleanup kit as described above, equivalent amounts of each fragment should be mixed to generate the reference standard.
3. The reference standard should be included in every capillary electrophoresis run. Afterward a standard curve should be prepared and used to interpolate the repeat number/AGG position.

4 Notes

1. Weigh 14.5 g $(NH_4)_2SO_4$ and add water to give a final volume of 50 ml, giving a 2.2 M solution. Filter through a 0.2 μM filter to sterilize. Store at room temperature. Do not substitute the commercially available "saturated" solutions.
2. Store the dNTPs in small aliquots at −20 °C and discard after three freeze–thaw cycles.
3. Make a 100 μM master stock of each primer by resuspension in the appropriate volume of 1× TE. Make up small volume

aliquots of 10 μM working stocks and store at −20 °C. Discard working stocks after three freeze–thaw cycles.

4. The previously published version of the assay [12] used Phusion® polymerase. However, subsequent tests showed that Q5® Hot Start polymerase gives a better fragment yield and eliminates the need to assemble the PCR reactions on ice. Due to their proofreading activity, these polymerases are not suitable for use in the AGG assay (but also *see* **Note 8**).
5. PstI, EcoRI, or Bsu36I restriction endonucleases can be substituted for HindIII.
6. Genomic DNA is stored at 4 °C in TE buffer at ~100 ng/μl. Significantly higher concentrations should not be used due to the difficulty of accurately pipetting small volumes of samples with high viscosity. Since adsorption to plasticware can reduce the amount of DNA in solution, the DNA concentrations should be based on a recent determination, preferably just prior to setting up the digestion reaction.
7. The two strands of the CGG-repeat containing PCR product do not migrate at the same rate and neither migrate at a rate consistent with their true size. Thus, for accurate repeat number determinations, a reference ladder of *FMR1* PCR products containing a known number of repeats and/or AGG interruptions should be used. A set of reference standards for both the Repeat PCR assay and the AGG PCR assays can be generated either directly from genomic DNA isolated from patient samples or, more sustainably, from patient cell lines or from cloned and sequence verified plasmid sequences (*see* Subheading 3.5). We have deposited two plasmids, 99255 and 99256, in the Addgene plasmid repository that can be used to prepare reference standards for both the Repeat PCR assay and the AGG PCR assay. Plasmid 99255 (aka pGLACTE-HT51-10) has the repeat structure: 9-A-9-A-78 and 99256 ((aka pGLACTE-HT51-13) has the repeat structure: 9-A-9-A-9 [13]. Thus, in the AGG PCR assay using the A-primer these two plasmids will produce fragments corresponding to 10, 20, 79, and 89 repeats. In the assay using the T-primer, fragments corresponding to 10 and 20 repeats will be generated [13]. Combined with two other plasmids (pGLACTE-23297 and pGLACTE-7306; available on request), these plasmids can also be used as a set of reference standards for the Repeat PCR assay to create a ladder containing 23, 29, 52, and 98 repeats. Genomic DNA containing larger alleles of known size can be used to generate larger reference standards. The reference standards should contain at least four fragments spanning the range of expected repeat sizes that have been amplified using the same labeled primer as the fragments to be analyzed. Note:

These plasmids are prone to contraction when grown at 37 °C. Upon receipt of the Addgene stab streak it out immediately and verify the insert size and AGG interruption pattern as described in Subheading 3.5, **step** 7.

8. Note that, while in our hands the Repeat PCR assay with Q5® polymerase is more robust, KAPA2G polymerase can also be used for this assay. This has the advantage of requiring a single thermostable polymerase for both assays. Furthermore, since we have found that the Repeat PCR assay with KAPA2G works better when the AGG PCR buffer is used, this further simplifies the workflow since the same buffer can be used for both the Repeat PCR assay and the AGG PCR assay. If capillary electrophoresis is going to be the method of analysis the KAPA2G polymerase in the AGG buffer gives the best fragment resolution; however, if agarose gel electrophoresis is to be used and/or considerable mosaicism is expected then Q5 polymerase in the Repeat PCR buffer with enhanced dNTP concentration will be more appropriate.
9. While not absolutely essential, in our experience the best results are obtained if the repeat or AGG PCR assay is carried out on freshly digested template.
10. The solutions involved are both dense (betaine, DMSO) and contain detergent. The volumes being added are relatively small. Thus, it is critical that pipettes are properly calibrated, that care is taken with the pipetting steps, and that the resultant solution is carefully but completely mixed.
11. The previously published version of the assay [12] used a 0.2 mM final dNTP concentration. We have found that increasing the final dNTP concentration to 0.45 mM significantly improves the yield of large alleles even when they are in the presence of smaller alleles. However, the yield of smaller alleles is reduced at this dNTP concentration. At dNTP concentrations even higher than this, the yield of all alleles is reduced. This improvement in yield is only seen using the Q5/Phusion polymerases and increasing the final dNTP concentration beyond 0.2 mM significantly reduces the final yield for the KAPA2G polymerase in the AGG buffer.
12. Addgene plasmid 99257 (aka pGLACTE-PseudoHT51 [13]) is used to produce an internal positive PCR control fragment in the A-primed AGG PCR assay. Note: These plasmids are prone to contraction when grown at 37 °C. Upon receipt of the Addgene stab streak it out immediately and verify the insert size and AGG interruption pattern as described in Subheading 3.5, **step** 7.
13. During development of the assay we tried HindIII digestion as an alternative to sonication and HaeII and a replacement for HpaII. However, HindIII digestion gave inconsistent results,

possibly due to the presence of the CGG-repeat within the fragment that affects the efficacy of denaturation, while HpaII was consistently more reliable than HaeII at producing complete digestion.

14. It is essential that sonication is efficient and that most fragments are less than 1 kb in size. Failure to sonicate effectively will lead to an overestimation of the degree of methylation.
15. Exposure to UV light damages DNA and should be avoided if possible. Large quantities of DNA can be visualized using the visible light stain Crystal Violet (1 μg/ml in 1× TAE buffer) [14] or, with greater sensitivity, the PrepOne Sapphire Blue Light system (EmbiTec).
16. Long CGG-repeat tracts are difficult to propagate stably in bacteria and are difficult to sequence using conventional sequencing strategies. Thus, the source of CGG repeats for cloning is best limited to genomic DNA with a single allele having 120 repeats or less.
17. The presence of the betaine and DMSO in the PCR reaction vastly increases the PCR error rate so the 23 PCR cycles are a compromise between generating enough product to be useful and minimizing the incorporation of errors.

References

1. Lozano R, Rosero CA, Hagerman RJ (2014) Fragile X spectrum disorders. Intractable Rare Dis Res 3(4):134–146
2. Usdin K, Woodford KJ (1995) CGG repeats associated with DNA instability and chromosome fragility form structures that block DNA synthesis in vitro. Nucleic Acids Res 23 (20):4202–4209
3. Pretto DI, Mendoza-Morales G, Lo J et al (2014) CGG allele size somatic mosaicism and methylation in FMR1 premutation alleles. J Med Genet 51(5):309–318
4. Yrigollen CM, Durbin-Johnson B, Gane L et al (2012) AGG interruptions within the maternal FMR1 gene reduce the risk of offspring with fragile X syndrome. Genet Med 14 (8):729–736
5. Latham GJ, Coppinger J, Hadd AG et al (2014) The role of AGG interruptions in fragile X repeat expansions: a twenty-year perspective. Front Genet 5(244)
6. Nolin SL, Glicksman A, Ersalesi N et al (2015) Fragile X full mutation expansions are inhibited by one or more AGG interruptions in premutation carriers. Genet Med 17(5):358–364
7. Nolin SL, Sah S, Glicksman A et al (2013) Fragile X AGG analysis provides new risk predictions for 45-69 repeat alleles. Am J Med Genet A 161A(4):771–778
8. Lokanga RA, Entezam A, Kumari D et al (2013) Somatic expansion in mouse and human carriers of fragile X premutation alleles. Hum Mutat 34(1):157–166
9. Zhou Y, Kumari D, Sciascia N et al (2016) CGG-repeat dynamics and FMR1 gene silencing in fragile X syndrome stem cells and stem cell-derived neurons. Mol Autism 7:42
10. Miller SA, Dykes DD, Polesky HF (1988) A simple salting out procedure for extracting DNA from human nucleated cells. Nucleic Acids Res 16(3):1215
11. Nolin SL, Ding XH, Houck GE et al (2008) Fragile X full mutation alleles composed of few alleles: implications for CGG repeat expansion. Am J Med Genet A 146A(1):60–65
12. Hayward BE, Zhou Y, Kumari D et al (2016) A set of assays for the comprehensive analysis of FMR1 alleles in the fragile X-related disorders. J Mol Diagn 18(5):762–774
13. Hayward BE, Usdin K (2017) Improved assays for AGG interruptions in fragile X premutation carriers. J Mol Diagn 19(6):828–835
14. Yang Y, Jung DW, Bai DG et al (2001) Counterion-dye staining method for DNA in agarose gels using crystal violet and methyl orange. Electrophoresis 22(5):855–859

Chapter 5

One-Step Generation of Seamless Luciferase Gene Knockin Using CRISPR/Cas9 Genome Editing in Human Pluripotent Stem Cells

Meng Li, Jack Faro Vander Stoep Hunt, Anita Bhattacharyya, and Xinyu Zhao

Abstract

Human pluripotent stem cells (hPSCs) offer powerful platforms for studying mechanisms of human diseases and for evaluating potential treatments. Genome editing, particularly the CRISPR/Cas9-based method, is highly effective for generating cell and animal models to study genetic human diseases. However, the procedure for generating gene-edited hPSCs is laborious, time consuming and unintentional genetic changes may confound the consequent experiments and conclusions. Here we describe one-step knockin of the NanoLuc luciferase gene (Nluc) to the fragile X syndrome gene, *FMR1*, in a human embryonic stem cell line (hESC), H1, and a fragile X disease model human induced pluripotent stem cell line (hiPSC), FX-iPSC. The luciferase reporter cell lines provide new platforms for exploring potential treatments for fragile X syndrome. The shortened and scarless targeting method described here can be effectively applied to other genes.

Key words Genome editing, CRISPR/Cas9, Knockin, Human pluripotent stem cells, *FMR1*, Fragile X, Luciferase reporter

1 Introduction

Human pluripotent stem cells offer great opportunities for studying human diseases, especially for modeling human diseases that are not recapitulated by animal models. Fragile X syndrome is caused by transcriptional silencing of *FMR1* gene that leads to loss of its coded protein, FMRP. The molecular mechanisms underlying *FMR1* silencing cannot be recapitulated in animal models. Fortunately, various fragile X human embryonic stem cell (hESC) and human induced pluripotent stem cell (hiPSC) lines have been generated for potential delineation of mechanisms of *FMR1* silencing and can be used to develop possible strategies to reactivate *FMR1* [1–4]. High-throughput screening (HTS) of compounds

Dalit Ben-Yosef and Yoav Mayshar (eds.), *Fragile-X Syndrome: Methods and Protocols*, Methods in Molecular Biology, vol. 1942, https://doi.org/10.1007/978-1-4939-9080-1_5,

for reactivation of *FMR1* have been performed but these antibody-based assays show poor sensitivity and are expensive and/or difficult to scale up [5, 6]. Luciferase-based HTS has been shown to be highly sensitive and can be scaled up [7]. Therefore, we created luciferase reporter lines of FX-iPSCs that have great potential for large-scale HTS of compounds to detect *FMR1* activation.

Genome editing is a critical tool for generating specific genetic models of diseases. However, previous genome editing methods, such as TALEN and ZFN, are technically challenging, necessitating expertise not common in most research laboratories. CRISPR/Cas9-based methods developed in the past few years are more efficient and more technically accessible, leading to a recent boom of genome editing of animals and cells for human disease modeling. Most of these studies involve gene knockdown through guide-RNA (sgRNA) guided Cas9 indel deletion. Gene-specific knockin is significantly more challenging and time-consuming, and therefore only limited laboratories have published data using this method.

Here we describe the one-step generation of luciferase reporter cell lines by knocking in an Nluc gene to the endogenous *FMR1* gene in *FMR1*-expressing H1 hESC line and *FMR1*-silenced FX-iPSC line. Our method can be adapted for knockin of fluorescent protein genes or drug-resistant genes to specific genomic loci. In our methods, cell lines with gene knockin can be obtained in about 4 weeks.

2 Materials

2.1 Construction of Plasmids for Gene Editing

1. Restriction enzymes BsmBI, BamHI, and NotI.
2. T4 DNA ligase.
3. AccuPrime Pfx DNA Polymerase (ThermoFisher).
4. Gibson Assembly Cloning Kit (New England Biolabs).

2.2 hPSC Culture

1. hEB media: 400 ml DMEM/F12, 100 ml Knockout serum replacement (KOSR) (ThermoFisher), 5 ml MEM NEAA, 2.5 ml L-glutamine, 3.5 μl 2-mercaptoethanol.
2. hESC media: hEB media supplemented with 6 ng/ml FGF-2.
3. Mouse embryonic feeders (MEFs).
4. 6-well plates and 24-well plates.
5. 1 mg/ml collagenase or dispase.

2.3 Electroporation of hPSCs and Temporary Puromycin Selection

1. 1–6 well plate of hPSCs at confluence ready for passaging.
2. 3–6 well plates of MEFs.
3. MEF-conditioned media: 24 h after plating MEFs, aspirate media and wash MEFs once with DMEM. Feed MEFs with

2 ml/well of hEB media. Next day collect the conditioned hEB media from the MEF wells to conical tubes labeled "MEF-conditioned hEB" and feed MEFs with fresh hEB media. Collect MEF-conditioned hEB media every day for 10 days. MEF-conditioned hEB media can be stored at 4 °C for 1 week or at −20 °C for 2 months. Add FGF-2 to MEF-conditioned hEB media to final concentration of 10 ng/ml to get MEF-conditioned hESC media and use within 1 week.

4. 10 mM ROCK inhibitor (Y-27632 dihydrochloride).
5. TrypLE express (ThermoFisher).
6. 4 mm electroporation cuvettes (Phenix Research Products) for use with Gene Pulser Xcell (Bio-Rad)
7. Puromycin.

2.4 Screening for Positive Colonies and Validation

1. Nano-Glo Luciferase Assay System (Promega).
2. QuickExtract DNA Extraction Solution (Epicentre).
3. EmeraldAmp GT PCR Master Mix (Takara).

2.5 Primers (Table 1)

Table 1
Custom DNA oligos should be dissolved in water to 25 μM

Name	Application	Sequence (5′-3′)
sgFMR1-F sgFMR1-R	sgRNA cloning	CACCGTAGGGTACTCCATTCACGAG AAACCTCGTGAATGGAGTACCCTAC
Green-F Green-R	Colony screening	ACTGAATCCTTGGTAACGAGACA CACCGCTCAGGACAATCCTT
P2A-F	Amplifying P2A-Nluc	TCTAGTTAACGGAGTACCCGCCACTAACTTCTCCCTGTTGA
Nluc-F		GCCACTAACTTCTCCCTGTTGAAACAAGCAGGGGATG TCGAAGAGAATCCTGGTCCAATGGTCTTCACAC TCGAAGATT
Nluc-R		CCATTCACTTACGCCAGAATGCGTTCGCACA
HA-L-F	Amplifying 5′ homology arm	TACCGAGCTCGGATCCACATGCACATACCCACTACTT
HA-L-R HA-R-F	Amplifying 3′ homology arm	ACTCCGTTAACTAGAGGTTGCTGACCATCCACGCTGTC ATTCTGGCGTAAGTGAATGGAGTACCCTAAACTGC
HA-R-R		CATGCTCGAGCGGCCACCTGCTTCCAATGTTTCTTAGAC

3 Methods

Maintenance and splitting of hPSCs should be performed as described [2, 8]. Six-well plates are used unless otherwise specified. In this method hPSCs are cultured on MEF feeder layer, but the method has been successfully applied to hPSCs grown on Matrigel (feeder-free).

3.1 Constructing Cas9-sgRNA Plasmid

1. Design and construct sgRNA plasmid (LentiCRISPR-sgRNA). sgRNA can be designed using published tools [9]. Clone sequences for expressing sgRNA into vector plasmid "lenti-CRISPR" (Addgene# 49535) as described previously [10, 11].
2. Digest vector plasmid with BsmBI overnight and purify the digested vector plasmid using column purification.
3. Anneal a pair of DNA oligos (*see* Table 1, sgFMR1-F and sgFMR1-R) at 1 μM each in 20 μl of 1× T4 DNA ligase buffer in a thermocycler with the following program: 95 °C 5 min, then cool down by 0.1 °C per second to 20 °C. Dilute the annealed oligos 1:100 with water.
4. Ligate 3 μl of the diluted oligos and 100 ng of the digested vector plasmid in 10 μl reaction solution containing 1× T4 DNA ligase buffer and 0.5 μl T4 DNA ligase at room temperature for 10 min.
5. Transform 2 μl of the ligation solution to competent *E. coli*. Screen positive plasmids by restriction mapping and validate by Sanger sequencing.

3.2 Constructing Nluc Donor Plasmid as Previously Described in Li et al. [12]

1. Digest vector plasmid Addgene# 31938 with BamHI and NotI.
2. PCR amplify homology arms (HA) and Nluc gene with Pfx DNA Polymerase using primers as below (*see* Table 1):

   5′ HA: HA-L-F and HA-L-R.
   3′ HA: HA-R-F and HA-R-R.
   Nluc: P2A-F, Nluc-F, and Nluc-R
3. Purify digested vector plasmid and PCR amplicons. Mix 100 ng of digested vector with equal moles of purified 5′ HA, 3′ HA, and Nluc in a 20 μl reaction solution containing 10 μl of 2× Gibson Assembly Master Mix. Incubate the solution at 50 °C for 60 min. Transform 2 μl of the solution to competent *E. coli*. Screen positive plasmids by restriction mapping and validate with Sanger sequencing.

3.3 Generating Knockin Lines with CRISPR/Cas9 and Donor Plasmid

In this study, we generate(d) luciferase reporter hPSC lines by knocking-in a Nluc gene to endogenous FMR1 gene using plasmids described in Subheadings 3.1 and 3.2 (Fig. 1).

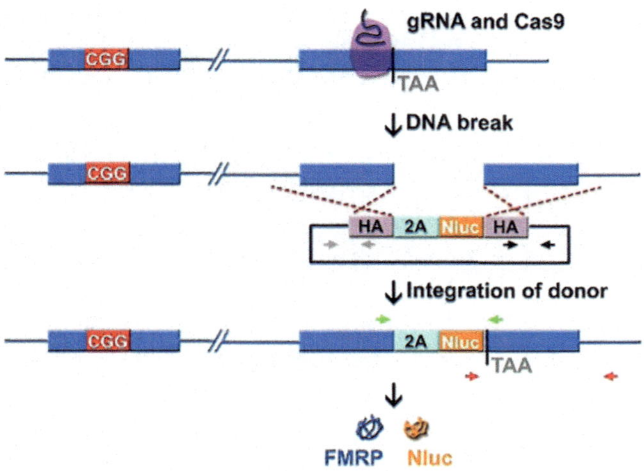

Fig. 1 Diagram of knockin of Nluc gene to endogenous *FMR1* gene by genome editing (Published in ref. 8)

1. Start with one plate of hPSCs that are at confluence for passaging and three MEF plates for plating cells after electroporation.
2. Change media on hPSCs to hESC media containing 10 μM ROCK inhibitor for >1 h prior to electroporation (*see* **Note 1**).
3. Aspirate media on hPSCs. Add 0.5 ml/well of TrypLE express and incubate in 37 °C incubator for 5–10 min. Aspirate TrypLE and add 2 ml/well of hESC media. Dissociate cells by gentle pipetting using P1000. Transfer cells to a 15 ml conical tube and centrifuge at 300 × *g* for 3 min (*see* **Note 2**). Aspirate supernatant.
4. Mix 0.6 ml of MEF-conditioned hESC media with plasmids (10 μg of Cas9-sgRNA plasmid and 15 μg donor plasmid). Use this mixture to resuspend hPSC cell pellet from last step by gentle pipetting with P1000. Transfer resuspended cells to a fresh electroporation cuvette.
5. Electroporate hPSCs in Gene Pulser Xcell with settings: 250 V, 500 μF, and resistance infinite. Electroporation time should be between 10 and 16 ms.
6. Gently transfer hPSCs from the cuvette into a 15 ml conical tube containing 9 ml of prewarmed MEF-conditioned hESC media supplemented with 10 μM ROCK inhibitor. Gently invert the tube once and incubate cells at 37 °C for 10 min (*see* **Note 3**).
7. While hPSCs incubate, prepare three plates of MEF feeders by aspirating media, washing once with DMEM, and adding 1.5 ml of MEF-conditioned hESC media supplemented with 10 μM ROCK inhibitor to each well.

8. Following the 10-min incubation, gently invert the tube with hPSCs once and plate 0.5 ml/well of cells to the three prepared MEF plates. Gently rock the plates a few times and put the plates in 37 °C incubator. Change media 24 h after electroporation to either regular hESC media or puromycin selection media (*see* next step).
9. For transient puromycin selection, change media on hPSCs daily with 2 ml/well of puromycin-containing MEF-conditioned media. For best results, apply different selection stringency to each plate as follows (*see* **Note 4**): plate #1: 0.5 μg/ml puromycin from 24 h after electroporation to 72 h after electroporation; plate #2: 0.5 μg/ml puromycin from 24–72 h then 0.25 μg/ml puromycin from 72–96 h; plate #3: 0.5 μg/ml puromycin from 24–96 h.
10. After puromycin selection, feed cells daily with MEF-conditioned media (preferred) or hESC media until colonies grow to the size similar to the size of colonies for regular passaging (about 2 weeks after electroporation). Keep the plate with 10–50 colonies per well and discard the plates with too many colonies (*see* **Note 5**).

3.4 Screening Colonies for Positive Knockin and Random Insertion

3.4.1 Picking Colonies

1. Mark and label colonies of good morphology (no obvious spontaneous differentiation) and median sizes (*see* **Note 6**). Also, choose colonies that are clearly separated from surrounding colonies and avoid mixed colonies.
2. Wash cells twice with hESC media to get rid of dead cells.
3. Scrape off half of a colony with P200 pipette and tips under a dissecting microscope and transfer the detached cells to PCR tubes [13].
4. Pick 24–48 colonies for initial screen and more if needed. For negative control, a couple of colonies of parental (WT) cell line should be collected at the same time.
5. Spin the PCR tubes for 15–30 s. Aspirate supernatant without disturbing cell pellet (fine to leave a few microliter of supernatant).
6. Perform colony screening for successful knockin (*see* Subheading 3.4.2). Within 2 days, transfer the other half of the positive colonies to a 24-well MEF plate (*see* Subheading 3.4.3).

3.4.2 Screening of Colonies for Positive Knockin of Nluc Gene

Here we describe two screening methods. H1 cells express *FMR1* therefore luciferase would also be expressed when Nluc gene is knocked in correctly. In such case luciferase activity assay should be performed as a quick way to screen for correct integration of Nluc gene (**step 1**). On the other hand, *FMR1* is silenced in FX-iPSCs and therefore PCR genotyping is used for screening (**step 2**).

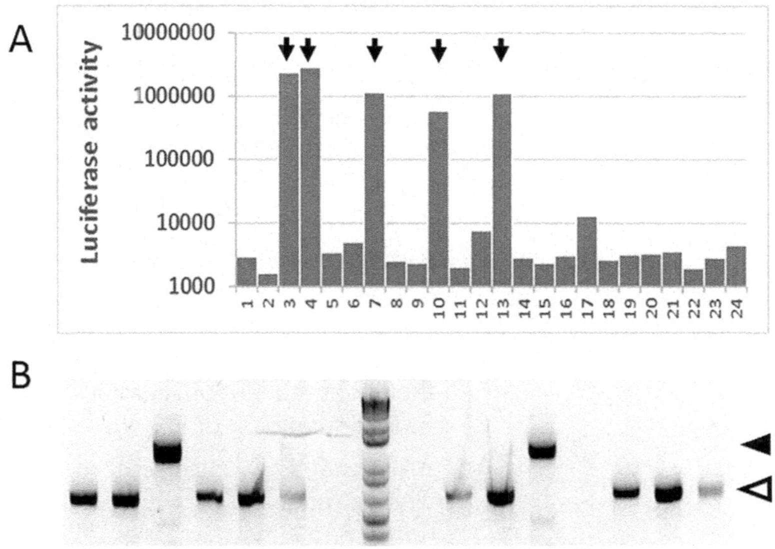

Fig. 2 Screening of colonies for positive knockin of Nluc gene. (**a**) Screening of H1 cells by luciferase activity assay. Positive colonies with high luciferase activities are indicated by arrowheads. (**b**) Screening of FX-iPSCs by genotyping. Positive colonies are indicated by solid arrowhead

1. Screening by Luciferase Assay
   (a) Add 25 μl of Nano-Glo Luciferase Assay solution (substrate–buffer 1:50) to cell pellet (**step 5** in Subheading 3.4.1).
   (b) Incubate for 5 min at room temperature then measure luminescence (Fig. 2a).
2. Screening by Genotyping
   (a) Add 20 μl of QuickExtract DNA Extraction Solution to cell pellet (**step 5** in Subheading 3.4.1) and resuspend cells by vortexing or pipetting up and down several times.
   (b) Put the PCR tubes in a thermocycler and run the following program: 60 °C 15 min, 65 °C 15 min, 98 °C 10 min, 4 °C hold (*see* **Note 7**).
   (c) After the program finishes, for each sample to be genotyped add 1 μl of the gDNA solution to 20 μl of solution containing 10 μl of EmeraldAmp GT PCR Master Mix and 0.16 μl of each primer Green-F and Green-R. Run the genotyping PCR in a thermocycler with the following program: 98 °C 2 min; 35 cycles of 98 °C 20 s, 58 °C 30 s, 72 °C 1 min 30s; 72 °C 5 min; 4 °C hold.
   (d) Separate the PCR amplicons on 2% agarose gel. Positive colonies are indicated by a higher band (solid arrowhead) due to knockin of Nluc gene (Fig. 2b).

3.4.3 Expanding Cells that Are Positive for Genome Editing (See ***Note 8****)*

1. Prepare a 24-well MEF plate. Aspirate MEF media, rinse once with DMEM, then add 0.5 ml/well of hESC media supplemented with 10 μM ROCK inhibitor.
2. Take out the 6-well plate with hPSCs positive for genome editing. Aspirate media and add 1 ml collagenase or dispase. Incubate at 37 °C for a period that is 1–2 min shorter than that for regular cell splitting.
3. Aspirate collagenase or dispase and add 2 ml hESC media. Scrape off the leftover half of positive hPSC colonies with P200 pipette and tips under a dissecting microscope and carefully transfer the cells to prepared 24-well MEF plates. Pick a desired number of cell colonies for secondary screening and/or further validation of genome editing.
4. After hPSCs have been picked to 24-well plate, break the cell clumps using P1000 set at 400 μl by pipetting gently up and down 3–5 times. Put the 24-well plate to incubator. Feed hESC media every day.

4 Notes

1. ROCK inhibitor can be added to hESC media the day before electroporation (~24 h treatment).
2. TrypLE digestion time should be empirically determined for individual cell lines. Cells should be easy to dissociate after digestion. If digestion time is longer than 5 min, gently rock plate once 5 min after adding TrypLE to avoid drying at the center of a well. Cells can also be dissociated in TrypLE (TrypLE is not aspirated after digestion), in which case, transfer cells suspended in TrypLE (3 ml) to a conical containing 12 ml of hESC media and invert to mix before centrifugation.
3. Incubating cells at 37 °C for 5–15 min before plating improves cell survival for some hPSC cell lines.
4. The puromycin selection conditions work for our cell lines. Conditions may need to be optimized for other cell lines.
5. Choose the plate that has the most individual colonies. If there are too many colonies, some colonies can be mixture from close colonies. Avoid those mixed colonies when picking for screening.
6. In our experience, cell colonies of median sizes that are closer to the center of the wells are more likely to be positive.
7. The gDNA solution can be stored at 4 °C for 1 week or − 20 °C for long-term storage.
8. Although in some protocols cell colonies are picked directly by scraping, in our experience, a gentle digestion before picking

helps with cell survival significantly, especially for some cell lines that are more difficult to culture.

9. The method described here has been used to create human FX reporter hPSC lines [12].

Acknowledgments

This work was supported by grants from the National Institutes of Health (R01MH078972 to X.Z, U54HD090256 to the Waisman Center), John Merck Fund (to X.Z and AB), Jenni and Kyle Professorship (to X.Z), and a Rath Graduate Fellowship to JH.

References

1. Avitzour M, Mor-Shaked H, Yanovsky-Dagan S et al (2014) FMR1 epigenetic silencing commonly occurs in undifferentiated fragile X-affected embryonic stem cells. Stem Cell Reports 3(5):699–706
2. Doers ME, Musser MTF, Nichol R, Nichol RF, Berndt ER et al (2014) iPSC-derived forebrain neurons from FXS individuals show defects in initial neurite outgrowth. Stem Cells Dev 23 (15):1777–1787
3. Eiges R, Urbach A, Malcov M et al (2007) Developmental study of fragile X syndrome using human embryonic stem cells derived from preimplantation genetically diagnosed embryos. Cell Stem Cell 1(5):568–577
4. Sheridan SD, Theriault KM, Reis SA et al (2011) Epigenetic characterization of the FMR1 gene and aberrant neurodevelopment in human induced pluripotent stem cell models of fragile X syndrome. PLoS One 6(10): e26203
5. Kaufmann M, Schuffenhauer A, Fruh I et al (2015) High-throughput screening using iPSC-derived neuronal progenitors to identify compounds counteracting epigenetic gene silencing in fragile X syndrome. J Biomol Screen 20(9):1101–1111
6. Kumari D, Swaroop M, Southall N et al (2015) High-throughput screening to identify compounds that increase fragile X mental retardation protein expression in neural stem cells differentiated from fragile X syndrome patient-derived induced pluripotent stem cells. Stem Cells Transl Med 4(7):800–808
7. Jang SW, Lopez-Anido C, MacArthur R et al (2012) Identification of drug modulators targeting gene-dosage disease CMT1A. ACS Chem Biol 7(7):1205–1213
8. Zhang SC, Wernig M, Duncan ID et al (2001) In vitro differentiation of transplantable neural precursors from human embryonic stem cells. Nat Biotechnol 19(12):1129–1133
9. http://crispr.mit.edu/. Accessed 16 Jan 2018
10. Shalem O, Sanjana NE, Hartenian E et al (2014) Genome-scale CRISPR-Cas9 knockout screening in human cells. Science 343 (6166):84–87
11. Debnath A, Parsonage D, Andrade RM et al (2012) A high-throughput drug screen for Entamoeba histolytica identifies a new lead and target. Nat Med 18(6):956–960
12. Li M, Zhao H, Ananiev GE et al (2017) Establishment of reporter lines for detecting fragile X mental retardation (FMR1) gene reactivation in human neural cells. Stem Cells 35 (1):158–169
13. Yusa K (2013) Seamless genome editing in human pluripotent stem cells using custom endonuclease-based gene targeting and the piggyBac transposon. Nat Protocols 8 (10):2061–2078

Chapter 6

Modeling FXS with Mouse Neural Progenitors

Ulla-Kaisa Peteri and Maija L. Castrén

Abstract

The neurosphere assay is a widely used method to culture neural precursor cells (NPCs), which include mixed populations of neural stem and progenitor cells, from the mammalian central nervous system. *Fmr1*-knockout (KO) mice generated to model fragile X syndrome (FXS) recapitulate the major phenotype of FXS. Neurosphere differentiation of cortical progenitors derived from brains of *Fmr1*-KO mice has been shown to reflect disordered mechanisms during cortical development in FXS in vivo. The cellular composition of neurospheres is heterogeneous, but robust FXS-specific alterations can be identified when culturing conditions are kept constant.

Key words Mouse, Cell culture, Brain, Neurosphere, Differentiation, Neural progenitor

1 Introduction

The neurosphere method to study neural progenitor cells (NPCs) was first described in 1992 by Reynolds and Weiss [1]. They cultured embryonic striatal cells in the presence of epidermal growth factor (EGF) and demonstrated formation of detached clusters of nestin-positive proliferating cells termed neurospheres. The culture conditions allowed enrichment and expansion of NPCs on the basis of their ability to self-renew over an extended time period and capacity to generate a large number of progeny although specific cell surface markers and stem cell morphology were lacking. Multilineage differentiation potential confirms the stem cell properties of NPCs in neurospheres [2].

Neurospheres consist of NPCs, including neural stem cells and progenitors [2, 3]. Cellular composition is heterogeneous and depends on the tissue source [4]. Mitogens stimulate cell proliferation and their withdrawal initiates differentiation of NPCs on coated matrix into different types of neuronal cells: neurons, astrocytes and oligodendrocytes [5]. Culture conditions, including mitogen exposure, cell density and number of passages, influence the cellular composition of neurospheres and differentiation of NPCs [6, 7].

Dalit Ben-Yosef and Yoav Mayshar (eds.), *Fragile-X Syndrome: Methods and Protocols*, Methods in Molecular Biology, vol. 1942, https://doi.org/10.1007/978-1-4939-9080-1_6,

Neurosphere assay has been used to study neurobiology of FXS neural progenitors [7–12]. Neural colony-forming cell assay [13] initially showed that the stem cell frequency did not differ in neurospheres derived from the embryonic brains of wild-type and *Fmr1*-knockout (KO) mice, the mouse model of FXS. FXS neurospheres display disease-specific features including increased differentiation of neural progenitors into transit-amplifying cells characterized in the developing brain of *Fmr1*-KO mice [14]. These transit-amplifying cells are not converted into neural stem cells in vitro [13]. In addition, functional analysis of FXS cortical progenitors revealed alterations of early differentiation of glutamate-responsive cells when compared with wild-type controls [11]. Altered glutamatergic signaling in FXS progenitors correlate with neurodevelopmental defects in FXS mouse brain, indicating that the neurosphere assay provides a method for modeling pathophysiology of FXS in vitro.

We describe the procedure for the culture of cortical progenitors from embryonic mouse brain at embryonic day 14 (E14). Neurosphere cultures can be expanded and neurospheres pooled for different types of experimental approaches. We provide instructions for cryopreservation as well as differentiation of neurospheres into neuronal cells, which allow for characterization of neural progenitor differentiation by immunohistochemistry, time-lapse and calcium imaging, and electrophysiology.

2 Materials

Reserve separate sets of microdissecting instruments for skin, embryo sac, and embryonic brain. Sterilize the dissection instruments by autoclaving or in antiseptic solution followed by sterile water, rinse and keep in 95% ethanol. Use disposable 70 μm nylon cell strainers for separation of single cells after dissociation of the tissues. Disinfect the dissection area with 70% ethanol. Diligently follow the waste disposal regulations when disposing waste materials.

Prepare all reagents, media, and supplements sterile, and handle them under aseptic conditions in a culture hood. Set the water bath to +37 °C.

2.1 Dissection Solutions

1. BSA–glucose–PBS: Dissolve 500 mg of BSA in 500 mL of PBS. Add 5 mL 1 M glucose and sterilize by filtration (0.2 μm). Store the solution at −20 °C.
2. Glucose, Hank's Balanced Salt Solution (HBSS), pH 7.5: Measure 5 mL HBSS, 1.5 mL 1 M glucose and 0.75 mL 1 M HEPES and add H_2O to a final volume of 50 mL. Sterile filter and store at +4 °C.

3. Sucrose-HBSS, pH 7.5: Dissolve 15.4 g sucrose in 45 mL of distilled H_2O in a 50 mL Falcon tube. Add 2.5 mL HBSS and make up to 50 mL with distilled H_2O. Sterile filter and store at +4 °C.
4. BSA, Earle's Balanced Salt Solution (EBSS), HEPES, pH 7.5: Dissolve 2 g BSA in 45 mL of EBSS in a 50 mL Falcon tube. Add 1 mL 1 M HEPES buffer and make up to 50 mL with EBSS. Sterile filter and store at +4 °C.
5. Dissociation buffer: Prepare the dissociation buffer fresh before use. Dissolve 66.5 mg trypsin, 35 mg hyaluronidase, 10 mg kynurenic acid in 50 mL HBSS-glucose solution. Sterile filter the solution and add 1 mL 4000 U/mL DNase. Warm up the buffer at +37 °C before starting the dissection. Prepare 5 mL of dissociation buffer for each brain.
6. Glucose stock solution: Dissolve 18.2 g glucose in 100 mL distilled H_2O. Sterile filter (0.2 μm) and store at −20 °C.

2.2 Growth Factors

1. 50 μg/mL epidermal growth factor (EGF): Prepare the stock solution by dissolving 50 μg of EGF in 1 mL of sterile H_2O.
2. 50 μg/mL basic fibroblastic growth factor (bFGF): Prepare the stock solution by dissolving 50 μg bFGF in 1 mL of sterile 5 mM Tris, pH 7.6.

The growth factors can be store at +4 °C for a week. For extended storage, add carrier protein (e.g., 0.1% BSA) and store the growth factors aliquoted at −20 °C to −80 °C. Avoid free-ze–thaw cycles.

2.3 Cell Culture Reagents

1. Neurosphere medium (NSM): DMEM/F12 supplemented with 1× B27 minus vitamin A, 1× penicillin–streptomycin, 2 mM L-glutamine, and 1 M HEPES. The medium can be stored at +4 °C for 2 weeks. Add mitogens before use for proliferating cell culture.
2. 2× Freezing medium: NMS, 20% dimethyl sulfoxide (DMSO), 40% FBS. Prepare 0.5 mL of freezing media per vial fresh before use.
3. 0.5 mg/mL poly-DL-ornithine: Dissolve 25 mg of poly-DL-ornithine in 50 mL PBS. Sterile-filter the solution and store at −20 °C.

3 Methods

3.1 Dissection of Embryonic Brains

1. Before beginning the dissociation, prepare all the solutions and preheat to +37 °C (*see* **Note 1**).
2. Pregnant mouse is euthanized by CO_2 asphyxiation and decapitated.

3. Lay the animal supine on absorbent pad and spray the abdominal skin with 70% ethanol. Pinch the skin with forceps and cut a small incision in the midline with surgical scissors. Expose the abdomen by pulling the skin apart toward the head and tail. Grasp the peritoneum with a second set of forceps and cut to expose the abdominal cavity. Locate the uterus and two uterine horns in the dorsal body cavity. Grasp the uterus below the oviduct and cut it free to remove the uterine horns. Place dissected uterus in ice cold BSA-glucose-PBS.
4. Grasp the muscular uterine lining and cut the muscle layer and decidua to expose each embryo. Collect the heads to BSA–glucose–PBS in the wells of a 96-well plate.
5. Dissect the brains from the head of mouse embryos using fine forceps. Carefully remove the skull with curved forceps and remove meninges under dissecting microscope (*see* **Note 2**).
6. Dissect the lateral wall of the lateral ventricles under a dissecting microscope and collect the tissue fragments of each brain separately to BSA–glucose–PBS in a 96-well plate.

3.2 Dissociation of Brain Tissue

1. Transfer the tissue fragments with a 5 mL pipette into preheated dissociation buffer containing trypsin, hyaluronidase, kynurenic acid, and DNase in a 5 mL conical tube. Incubate in a water bath at +37 °C for 15 min, triturate gently 10 times with 5 mL pipette and continue incubation for additional 15 min.
2. Pass the dissociated tissue through a 70 μm nylon cell strainer.
3. Centrifuge the cells at 200 × *g* for 5 min in a 15 mL conical tube, remove supernatant, and resuspend the pellet in 4 mL Sucrose-HBSS.
4. Centrifuge the cell suspension at 250 × *g* for 10 min, remove supernatant, and resuspend pellet in 2 mL 1× EBSS.
5. Fill a set of new 15 mL conical tubes with 12 mL BSA-EBSS-HEPES-solution. Carefully apply the cell suspension to the top and centrifuge for 7 min at 200 × *g*.
6. Remove supernatant and resuspend in 0.5 mL of NSM. Calculate the viable cell concentration with a hematocytometer and plate cells at the density of 50,000–100,000 cells/mL. Add bFGF and EGF to the culture medium at the final concentration of 10 ng/mL and 20 ng/mL, respectively.
7. Cultures are maintained at +37 °C in a humidified atmosphere containing 5% CO_2. Neurospheres of variable size (50–100 μm) will form in the culture within a week (Fig. 1).

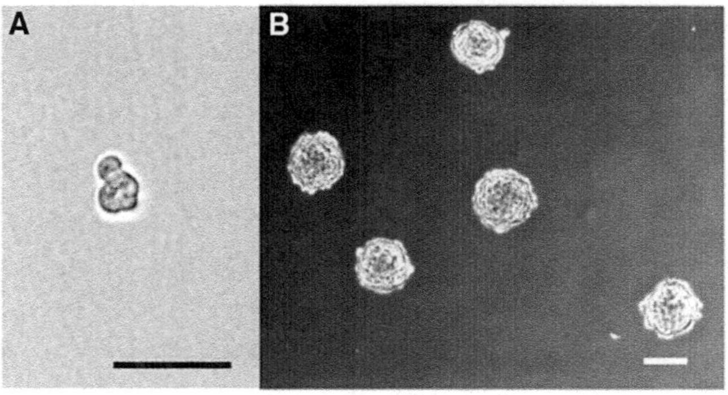

Fig. 1 (**a**) Initiation of neurosphere formation within first hours and (**b**) after 10 days in culture

3.3 Neurosphere Culture

3.3.1 Medium Change

1. Medium change is performed twice a week and the growth factors are added three times per week (*see* **Note 3**).
2. To change the medium, collect neurosphere suspension in a 15 mL falcon tube and harvest the cells at 200 × *g* for 5 min.
3. Replace half of the medium with fresh NSM. Add growth factors to the final concentrations of 20 ng/mL EGF and 10 ng/mL bFGF upon medium change (*see* **Note 4**).

3.3.2 Passaging Neurospheres

1. Neurospheres can be dissociated for the first time after harvesting the cells between days 5 and 9 when the cell cluster size starts to exceed an average of 350 μm.
2. Collect neurosphere suspension in a 15 mL Falcon tube and allow cells to settle down for approximately 10–15 min.
3. Reduce medium to 2 mL and dissociate cells manually by gently pipetting up and down (about ten times) using fire polished Pasteur pipette until the medium is clear and no cell clusters are visible (*see* **Note 5**).
4. Centrifuge at 200 × *g* for 5 min and remove the medium.
5. Resuspend cell pellet in 0.5 mL of fresh medium and calculate the viable cell concentration. Plate cells at the density of 100,000 cells/mL in NSM containing EGF and bFGF (*see* **Note 6**).
6. Repeat the dissociation of neurospheres approximately every 7–9 days (**steps 1–5**) (*see* **Note 7**).

3.4 Cryopreserving Neurospheres

3.4.1 Freeze Procedure

1. Harvest the neurospheres at 200 × *g* for 5 min.
2. Remove the media and carefully resuspend the cells in NSM. Add freezing media in 1:1 ratio and transfer 1 mL of cell suspension per cryovial (*see* **Note 8**).
3. Freeze the cells overnight in a freezing container at −80 °C.
4. On the following day, transfer the vials to liquid nitrogen for extended storage.

3.4.2 Thaw Procedure

1. Quickly thaw the neurospheres in +37 °C water bath. Wipe the vial with ethanol and transfer the cells to the laminar hood (*see* **Note 9**).
2. Pipette the cells into a 15 mL Falcon containing 5–10 mL of media.
3. Centrifuge at 200 × *g* for 5 min.
4. Remove the media and resuspend neurospheres in NSM containing EGF and bFGF.
5. Plate the neurospheres on a 10 cm dish in the final volume of 10 mL of media per well.

3.5 Neurosphere Differentiation

1. Before plating the cells, prepare poly-DL-ornithine-coated plates (*see* **Note 10**).
2. Dilute poly-DL-ornithine stock solution at 1:100 in PBS.
3. Coat the culture plates with approximately 0.15 mL/cm^2 of diluted poly-DL-ornithine.
4. Incubate the plates for 4 h to o/n at +37 °C.
5. Wash the plates three times with PBS or sterile H_2O. Do not let the coating dry.
6. For differentiation, transfer medium-sized neurospheres (200–250 μm) on the coated plates with NSM. Do not add the mitogens in the medium (*see* **Note 11**).
7. Cells migrated from the neurospheres within the first 24 h express early neuronal markers (*see* Fig. 2) (*see* **Note 12**).

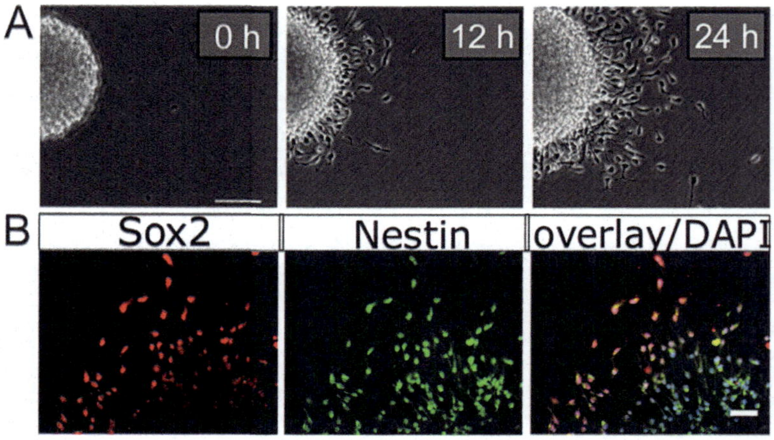

Fig. 2 (**a**) Neurosphere differentiation within 24 h period. (**b**) Immunostaining of cells migrated from the neurosphere 24 h after plating for the expression of Sox2 and Nestin. Scale bar, 100 μm (**a**), 50 μm (**b**)

4 Notes

1. Embryonic brains are dissected from a litter (between 7 and 16 pups) of a pregnant mouse. Each brain will be processed separately and the procedure has to be adjusted for an appropriate number of brains.
2. Excess brain tissue and cultured progenitors can be used for genotyping.
3. The growth factors are not stable at +37 °C and should be replenished regularly. It is sufficient to supplement EGF and bFGF when changing the medium and once more in between the medium changes by adding the growth factors directly to the culture dishes.
4. Do not change all of the medium at once. Factors secreted by neurospheres promote the growth and survival of the cells.
5. Alternatively a 1 mL mechanical pipette can be used. In this case, resuspend the cells in 0.5 to 1 mL of NSM. When pipetting the neurospheres, place the pipette tip at the bottom of the tube slightly tilted. Smaller opening at the end of the tip breaks the cell clusters more efficiently.
6. When pipetting cells for counting and plating, let the suspension settle for few minutes and collect the cells from the upper part of the suspension. In this way you will not collect the bigger cell clusters and debris that will settle to the bottom of the tube.
7. The neurospheres should be passaged when the cell cluster size starts to exceed 350–400 μm. If the neurospheres grow too big, the cells in the center start to turn necrotic which is visible under the microscope as darker area within the spheres.
8. In general, cells cultured in a 10 cm dishes can be cryopreserved in one vial. Avoid freezing a low number of neurospheres per vial because low cell density has a detrimental effect on cell survival.
9. Take the vial from the water bath when a small cluster of ice is still visible. Do not wait for the whole cell suspension to thaw as DMSO is toxic to cells and should be diluted rapidly.
10. Add the cover glasses when needed for later experiments.
11. Alternatively, neurospheres can be dissociated and cells plated as single cells on coated plates.
12. With extended culturing, the progenitors will mature into a heterogeneous population of neuronal cells.

Acknowledgments

This protocol was adapted from the method described by Johansson et al. [2] and our previously published paper [8]. This work was supported by Academy of Finland, Tuulikki and Sakari Sohlberg Foundation, and Arvo and Lea Ylppö Foundation.

References

1. Reynolds B, Weiss S (1992) Generation of neurons and astrocytes from isolated cells of the adult mammalian nervous system. Science 255:1707–1710
2. Johansson C, Momma S, Clarke D, Risling M, Lendahl U, Frisén J (1999) Identification of a neural stem cell in the adult mammalian central nervous system. Cell 96:25–34
3. Bez A, Corsini E, Curti D, Biggiogera M, Colombo A, Nicosia R, Pagano S, Parati E (2003) Neurosphere and neurosphere-forming cells: morphological and ultrastructural characterization. Brain Res 993:18–29
4. Maslov A, Barone T, Plunkett R, Pruitt S (2004) Neural stem cell detection, characterization, and age-related changes in the subventricular zone of mice. J Neurosci 24:1726–1733
5. Vescovi A, Reynolds B, Fraser D, Weiss S (1993) bFGF regulates the proliferative fate of unipotent (neuronal) and bipotent (neuronal/astroglial) EGF-generated CNS progenitor cells. Neuron 11(5):951–966
6. Suslov O, Kukekov V, Ignatova T, Steindler D (2002) Neural stem cell heterogeneity demonstrated by molecular phenotyping of clonal neurospheres. Proc Natl Acad Sci U S A 99:14506–14511
7. Sourial M, Doering L (2016) Astrocyte-secreted factors selectively Alter neural stem and progenitor cell proliferation in the fragile X mouse. Front Cell Neurosci 10:126
8. Castren M, Tervonen T, Karkkainen V, Heinonen S, Castren E, Larsson K, Bakker CE, Oostra BA, Akerman K (2005) Altered differentiation of neural stem cells in fragile X syndrome. Proc Natl Acad Sci U S A 102:17834–17839
9. Guo W, Allan AM, Zong R, Zhang L, Johnson EB, Schaller EG, Murthy AC, Goggin SL, Eisch AJ, Oostra BA, Nelson DL, Jin P, Zhao X (2011) Ablation of Fmrp in adult neural stem cells disrupts hippocampus-dependent learning. Nat Med 17:559–565
10. Louhivuori V, Vicario A, Uutela M, Rantamäki T, Louhivuori LM, Castrén E, Tongiorgi E, Akerman KE, Castrén ML (2011) BDNF and TrkB in neuronal differentiation of Fmr1-knockout mouse. Neurobiol Dis 41:469–480
11. Achuta VS, Grym H, Putkonen N, Louhivuori V, Kärkkäinen V, Koistinaho J, Roybon L, Castren ML (2017) Metabotropic glutamate receptor 5 responses dictate differentiation of neural progenitors to NMDA-responsive cells in fragile X syndrome. Dev Neurobiol 77:438–453
12. Sourial M, Doering L (2017) Abnormal neural precursor cell regulation in the early postnatal fragile X mouse hippocampus. Brain Res 1666:58–69
13. Louis S, Rietze R, Deleyrolle L, Wagey R, Thomas T, Eaves A, Reynolds B (2008) Enumeration of neural stem and progenitor cells in the neural colony-forming cell assay. Stem Cells 26:988–996
14. Tervonen TA, Louhivuori V, Sun X, Hokkanen ME, Kratochwil CF, Zebryk P, Castren E, Castren ML (2009) Aberrant differentiation of glutamatergic cells in neocortex of mouse model for fragile X syndrome. Neurobiol Dis 33:250–259

Chapter 7

Using Human Neural Progenitor Cell Models to Conduct Large-Scale Drug Screens for Neurological and Psychiatric Diseases

Jack Faro Vander Stoep Hunt, Meng Li, Xinyu Zhao, and Anita Bhattacharyya

Abstract

High-throughput drug screen (HTS) has become a viable approach for new treatment discovery in human diseases. Advances in gene editing technology and human pluripotent stem cell differentiation techniques have expanded the capability of HTS to identify potential treatments for human diseases of the central nervous system. Here, we describe techniques to use a human patient-derived neural progenitor cell luciferase reporter line to screen a large small molecule library.

Key words Drug screen, Large scale, Luciferase reporter, Neural progenitor cells, Human stem cells, Induced pluripotent stem cells

1 Introduction

High-throughput drug discovery has been successfully used to identify new treatments for human diseases including *Entamoeba hisolytica* infection [1], breast cancer [2], and secretory diarrhea [3]. Discovery of new treatments for neurological and psychiatric diseases via high-throughput cell-based screening methods has been hampered in part by two factors: (1) human specific pathogenesis that precludes use of animal cell models and (2) inaccessibility of primary human neural cells. With advances in gene-editing technology and human pluripotent stem cell (hPSC) differentiation techniques, the ability to use in vitro "disease in a dish" models to conduct large-scale, high-throughput drug screens to find new treatments for neurological and psychiatric diseases has greatly expanded. hPSCs can be derived from human patients and modified using CRISPR/Cas9 gene-editing to insert reporter genes for screening purposes [4]. Furthermore, hPSCs can be differentiated to neural progenitor cells (hNPCs) using established methods

Dalit Ben-Yosef and Yoav Mayshar (eds.), *Fragile-X Syndrome: Methods and Protocols*, Methods in Molecular Biology, vol. 1942, https://doi.org/10.1007/978-1-4939-9080-1_7,

[4, 5]. hNPCs are an attractive cell type to use in high throughput drug screens since they are readily proliferative, can be expanded to scale and can be differentiated to a number of cell types in the neural lineage for secondary screening purposes.

In the current chapter, we discuss the materials and methods necessary to: (1) differentiate hNPCs from hPSCs, (2) maintain, freeze and thaw hNPCs in culture, and (3) optimize conditions for scale-up of large-scale drug screen using hPSC-derived hNPCs and a luciferase-based reporter system. This methodology is dependent on the creation of hPSC reporter lines from patients with psychiatric or neurological diseases, which is not discussed in the present chapter.

2 Materials

2.1 Media Recipes

All components should be sterile and of tissue culture grade. Store reagents as suggested by the manufacturer, unless otherwise stated in protocol.

1. hESC media: 400 mL DMEM/F12, 100 mL Knockout Serum Replacement (Thermo Fisher), 5 mL 100× nonessential amino acids, 2.5 mL 100× L-glutamine. Combine the first 4 components and filter through 0.22 μm pore membrane. Add 4 ng/mL human recombinant FGF2 (*see* **Note 1**).
2. Chemically defined media: 50 mL DMEM/F12 media, 50 mL Neurobasal media, 2 mL B27 without vitamin A supplement (Thermo Fisher), 1 mL N2 supplement, 10uM SB432542, 100 nM LDN193189 (*see* **Note 1**).
3. Basal NPC media: 500 mL Neurobasal media, 5 mL 100× GlutaMAX (Thermo Fisher), 5 mL 100× Antibiotic-Antimycotic (Thermo Fisher), 5 mL N2 supplement, 10 mL B27 without vitamin A supplement (Thermo Fisher). Combine all components. Do not filter after adding N2 or B27 supplements. Use within 2 weeks.
4. Complete NPC media: Basal NPC media, 10 ng/mL final concentration FGF2 (*see* **Note 1**). Combine components and use within 1 week.
5. Passaging NPC media: Basal NPC media, 1 μg/mL final concentration Y-27632 dihydrochloride, 10 ng/mL final concentration FGF2 (*see* **Note 1**). Combine all components and use the same day.
6. Plating NPC media: Cold basal NPC media, 1 μg/mL final concentration Y-27632 dihydrochloride, 10 ng/mL final concentration FGF2 (*see* **Note 1**). Combine all components and keep on ice. Right before use, add 0.05 mg/mL final concentration Matrigel Matrix (Corning, *see* **Note 2**).

7. Matrigel coating media: Add 0.05 mg/mL final concentration Matrigel (Corning) to cold DMEM by using P1000 to transfer 1 mL cold DMEM between Matrigel aliquot and 50 mL conical of DMEM. Once Matrigel is completely thawed using this technique, transfer remaining Matrigel to cold DMEM (*see* **Note 2**).
8. Freezing NPC media: 10% DMSO, 90% Passaging NPC media.

2.2 Other Reagents and Supplies

1. TrypLE Express (Thermo).
2. Nano-Glo Luciferase Assay System (Promega).
3. Collagenase IV.
4. White, clear bottom 1536-well tissue culture microplate (Greiner).
5. White, clear bottom 386-well tissue culture microplate.
6. White, clear bottom 96-well tissue culture microplate.
7. 10 cm round tissue culture dishes.
8. Sealing Films (Axygen).

3 Methods

All procedures are performed under sterile conditions in a certified biosafety cabinet. All cells should be maintained in a HEPA-filtered cell incubator (37 °C, 5% CO_2).

3.1 Preparation of Matrigel-Coated Plates

1. Prepare aliquots of Matrigel using manufacturer's instructions and store at −80 °C. 0.5 mg of Matrigel is added to 10 mL DMEM to coat each 10 cm plate.
2. Aliquot 10 mL cold DMEM per 10 cm plate in sterile 50 mL conical tube. Keep tube on ice.
3. Remove appropriate Matrigel aliquot from −80 °C and immediately place on ice.
4. Add Matrigel to cold DMEM by using P1000 to transfer 1 mL cold DMEM between Matrigel aliquot and 50 mL conical. Once Matrigel is completely thawed using this technique, transfer remaining Matrigel to cold DMEM (*see* **Note 2**).
5. Quickly add 10 mL prepared cold Matrigel coating media to sterile round 10 cm tissue culture dish.
6. Leave plate at room temperature, for 1 h, without disturbing, to allow Matrigel to polymerize. After this, plates can be stored in cell incubator, 37 °C for up to 5 days before use.

3.2 Neural Differentiation to Create NPC Line

Detailed methods for hPSC culture and differentiation to hNPCs are described elsewhere [4, 5]. Brief methods are presented below.

1. Maintain hPSC line as colonies on MEF feeder layer with daily replacement of hESC media.
2. Passage hPSC colonies using 1 mg/mL collagenase IV in DMEM at least once per week. Some hPSC lines will grow more quickly and may need to be passaged more frequently.
3. Before NPC differentiation, prepare Matrigel-coated 10 cm plate(s).
4. For differentiation to NPCs, dissociate confluent hPSCs to single-cell suspension using TrypLE, wash and plates 500,000–1000,000 cells/cm^2 on Matrigel-coated plates in MEF-conditioned hESC media supplemented with 10 ng/ mL human recombinant FGF2 and 10 μM Y-27632 dihydrochloride.
5. The following day, cells should be nearly confluent. Induce neural differentiation by changing media to chemically defined media.
6. Culture cells for 10 days with daily change of chemically defined media.
7. Passage cells using TrypLE and culture on Matrigel-coated plates in complete NPC media (*see* Subheading 3.4 for more detail on this step).
8. NPCs will be ready for to test for screening procedure after five passages.

3.3 Daily NPC Maintenance

1. Grow NPCs on 10 cm plates in 10 mL of complete NPC media.
2. Check NPCs daily under microscope for morphology and confluency. Cells should have a roughly triangular shape and grow in small rosette-like clusters (Fig. 1a).

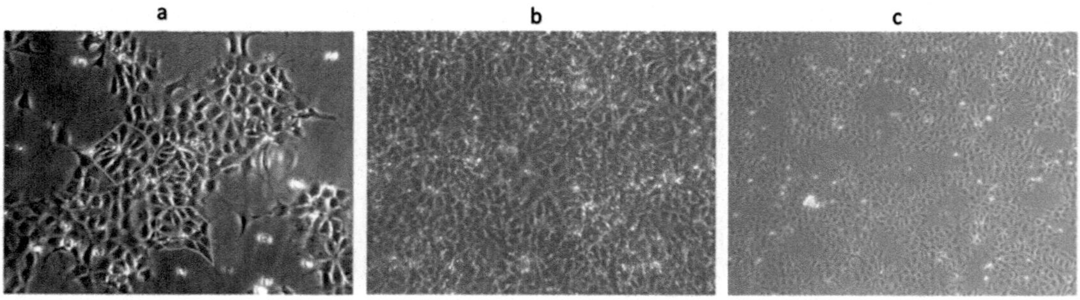

Fig. 1 (**a**) hNPCs at ~60–70% confluence growing with characteristic triangular morphology (20× magnification). Teal outline marks rosette-like structure characteristic of clusters of proliferating hNPCs. (**b**) hNPCs at 100% confluence, note more compact morphology of individuals cells as density increases (10× magnification). (**c**) hNPCs 24 h after passaging cells at 1:3 density (4× magnification)

3. Remove media and replace with fresh complete NPC media on day 1 after passaging (passaging = day 0).
4. From day 3 onward (day 2 can be skipped), media should be replaced daily, with complete NPC media, until next passage.

3.4 Passaging NPCs

1. Passage NPCs once they are 95–100% confluent (Fig. 1b).
2. Before passaging, prepare sufficient number of Matrigel-coated 10 cm dishes.
3. Remove media from NPCs and add 1 mL TrypLE Express. Tilt plate back and forth to ensure contact across entire plate surface.
4. Incubate at 37 °C, 5% CO_2. Every minute, remove the 10 cm dishes, tilt back and forth and check for first signs of cell detachment (usually apparent at edges of plate first). Once cells have just begun to detach, proceed to next step (*see* **Note 3**).
5. Add 4 mL DMEM to the dishes and use pipette to gently blow off all attached cells from the dishes.
6. Transfer cell suspension to a 15 mL conical tube.
7. Centrifuge at 300 × *g*, 3.5 min to pellet cells.
8. Aspirate all media.
9. Centrifuge at 300 × *g*, 15 s, remove any remaining TrypLE media using P200 (*see* **Note 4**).
10. Add 1 mL passaging NPC media to tube and triturate cells using P1000 to resuspend pellet.
11. Passage resuspended NPCs at a 1:3 ratio and plate in 10 mL passaging NPC media in new 10 cm dish. (Figure 1c shows NPCs passaged at 1:3 ratio on day 1 after passaging.)
12. The cells will be ready to passage again in ~3–4 days.

3.5 Freezing NPCs

1. NPCs can be frozen when they are 100% confluent.
2. Follow instructions in Subheading 3.4 through **step 8**.
3. Add 1 mL freezing NPC media and gently triturate using P1000 to resuspend pellet.
4. Add 2 mL additional freezing NPC media, mix and aliquot 1 mL into three labelled 2.0 mL screw cap cryovials.
5. Freeze cells in freezing container at −80 °C (*see* **Note 5**).
6. After 24 h, transfer freezing tubes to a liquid nitrogen storage container for long-term storage (*see* **Note 6**).

3.6 Thawing NPCs

1. To thaw NPCs, prepare Matrigel-coated plate (*see* Subheading 3.1) before thawing.
2. Aliquot 10 mL of basal NPC media into a 15 mL conical tube and warm for 15 min in 37 °C water bath.

3. Remove 1 cryovial of NPCs from liquid nitrogen storage.
4. Quickly thaw NPCs by gently swirling cryovial in 37 °C water bath. Check tube briefly every 30 s and remove as soon as cells have thawed completely.
5. Use P1000 to transfer NPCs dropwise into prewarmed basal NPC media while gently flicking tube.
6. Let NPCs settle for 1 min, gently invert tube.
7. Centrifuge at 300 × *g*, 3.5 min.
8. Aspirate all media from NPC pellet.
9. Resuspend NPC pellet in 1 mL passaging NPC media with gentle trituration.
10. Aspirate Matrigel coating media from 10 cm plate, add thawed NPCs in a final volume of 10 mL passaging NPC media.

3.7 Optimizing Culture Conditions for Large Scale Screen

All conditions can be optimized in 96-well plates for convenience and then scaled up to 384- or 1536-well format. This is one of the most important steps to ensure success in a large-scale drug screen, but requires an empiric approach and extensive optimization depending on the specific cell line and assay being used. General guidelines for a systematic approach to optimization are provided but specifics must be determined on a case-by-case basis.

1. Determine optimal length of drug treatment using 96-well format. This will vary, depending on assay and positive control being used, but should reflect the physiological process being studied. Ensure adequate time for gene transcription, translation, signal transduction, cell migration, adhesion, etc.
2. Determine optimal cell density. Optimal cell density will depend on the assay. NPC proliferation will decrease as plate becomes more confluent, presumably from contact inhibition and depletion of nutrients from media more quickly, so assays dependent on cell division/proliferation will likely need sparser cell density at initial plating. Reasonable starting cell number for various multiwell plates are as follows: 10,000–100,000 cells/well for 96-well format, 2000–20,000 cells/well for 386-well format, 1000–5000 cells/well for 1536-well format (*see* **Note 7**).
3. Scale to 384- or 1536-well format, using proportionally lower plating density dependent on surface area of plates. Optimal density may not scale linearly, so you will need to fine-tune the optimal cell density for each plate format.
4. Regularly check system for consistency. After thawing cells, passage at least three times and then test cells for adequate assay response in 96-well format before using for drug screen (*see* **Note 8**).

3.8 Conducting Primary Screen

Individual assay parameters will have to be determined before starting a large-scale screen. The example below is taken from a system using a Nano-Luciferase gene expression reporter cell line [4].

1. Prepare 40 mL passaging NPC media per 10 cm dish of NPCs and 2 mg Matrigel per 10 cm dish of NPCs and keep on ice until the time of plating. Do not add Matrigel to passaging NPC media until just before plating. Place 5 μL BioTek metal-tipped fluid dispensing cassette in refrigerator to chill before use (*see* **Note 2**).
2. Prepare NPCs from confluent 10 cm plates by following **steps 1–8** of Subheading 3.4 (Fig. 2, Step 1).
3. Resuspend NPCs in 2 mL prewarmed complete NPC media per 10 cm plate.
4. Count cells using hemacytometer or automated cell counter.
5. Prepare MicroFlo Select dispenser with prechilled 5 μL BioTek metal-tipped fluid dispensing cassette.
6. Add ice-cold Matrigel to cold passaging NPC media, shake to mix and return to ice.
7. Right before plating, add prepared NPC suspension to Matrigel/passaging NPC media mixture to a final concentration of 0.3×10^6 cells/mL, on ice (Fig. 2, Step 2, *see* **Note 9**). Gently invert several times to mix.
8. Dispense 5 μL cell mixture/well to a 1536-well clear bottom, white sided tissue culture plate using microscale fluid dispensing machine while gently and continuously swirling the tube containing NPC suspension on ice to mix (Fig. 2, Step 3). Mixing during plating will allow for more homogenous dispensing of NPC suspension across multiple plates.
9. Seal the plate with sealing film, return the plate to incubator. Allow at least 8 h for adequate cell attachment before adding compounds.
10. Add negative control (DMSO in example), positive control (5-aza-2′-deoxycytidine in example) and test compounds from premade 1536-well plates using Echo 550 to dispense nanoscale volumes (Fig. 2, Step 4).
11. Seal the plate with sealing film.
12. Incubate at 37 °C, 5% CO_2 for 72 h.
13. Prepare NanoGlo Reagent per manufacturer's instruction.
14. Add 5 μL NanoGlo Reagent/well using microscale fluid dispenser (Fig. 2, Step 5).
15. Incubate for 15 min, at room temperature.
16. Centrifuge at $80 \times g$, 1 min.

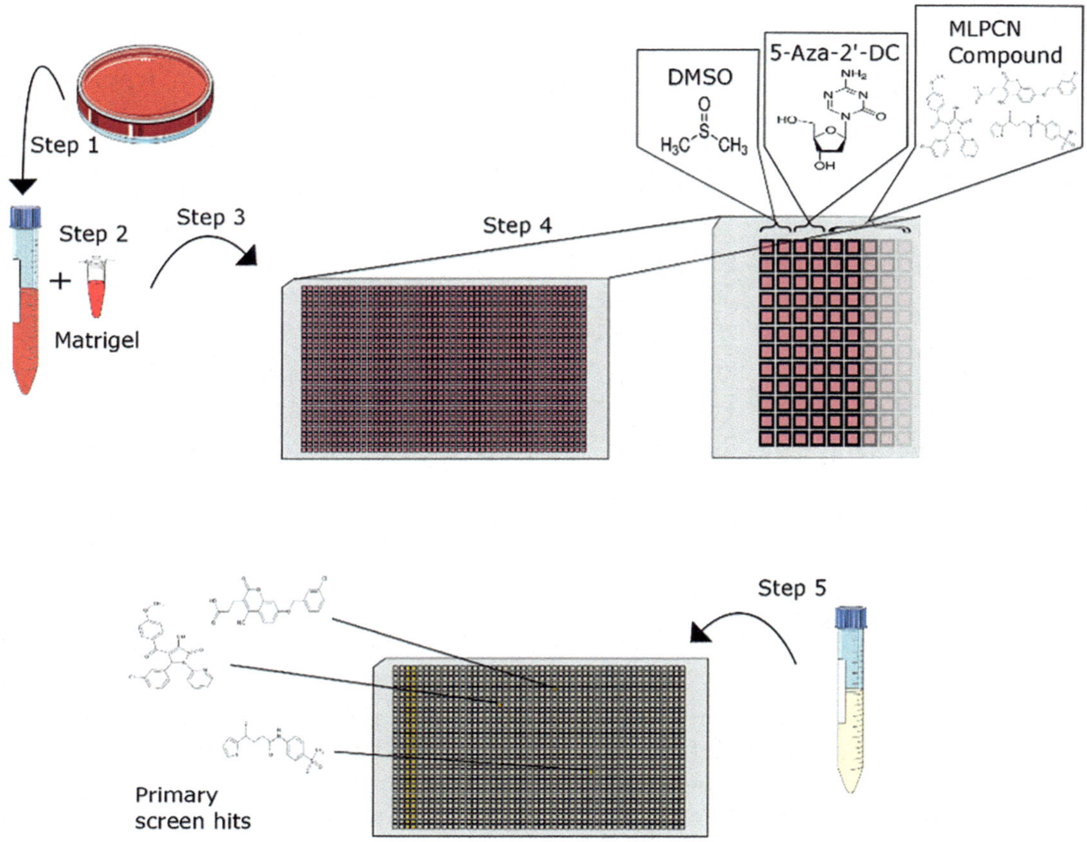

Fig. 2 Step 1. Dissociation of hNPCs growing on 10 cm plate. Step 2. Combination of cell suspension and Matrigel matrix, keeping all reagents on ice. Step 3. Plating cell–Matrigel suspension onto 1536-well plate using microscale fluid dispenser. Step 4. Adding test compounds from premade 1536-well plates using nanoscale fluid transfer machine. Step 5. Adding NanoGlo Reagent and reading luminescence on plate reader

17. Read luminescence on Pherastar plate reader or similar.
18. If only one replicate of each compound is used for screening, hits can be determined by the following formulas:

$$z' = 1 - 3 \times \frac{\sigma\text{PositiveCtl} + \sigma\text{NegativeCtl}}{|\mu\text{PositiveCtl-}\mu\text{NegativeCtl}|}$$

$$z = \frac{\text{SampleRLU-}\mu\text{NegativeCtl}}{\sigma\text{NegativeCtl}}$$

19. If an individual compound exceeds the minimum Z value, and its test plate exceeds minimum Z', the compound is deemed a hit on the primary screen (*see* **Note 10**).

4 Notes

1. FGF2, SB432542, LDN193189 and Y-27632 dihydrochloride are sensitive to freeze-thaw cycles and will lose efficacy if kept in reconstituted liquid form. Aliquot reconstituted molecules and store at −80 °C. Use thawed aliquots immediately (Y-27632 dihydrochloride) or within 1 week (FGF2, SB432542, LDN193189). Do not filter media after adding any of these compounds.
2. Matrigel Matrix must be kept as cold as possible at all times before plating. It will begin to polymerize and form a gel above 10 °C. Following the suggested procedure in Subheading 2.1 will prevent premature polymerization. In biosafety cabinet, prepare one-time use aliquots of Matrigel using manufacturer's instructions and store at −80 °C. 0.5 mg of Matrigel is needed per 10 mL of media, which is sufficient to coat one 10 cm^2 plate.
3. Stop incubation in TrypLE before cells are completely detached to increase cell viability. Cells should just be beginning to detach when you dilute TrypLE with DMEM.
4. This step is important as even a small amount of TrypLE left in the culture media can reduce NPC viability significantly.
5. Freezing container should ensure gradual cooling of −1 °C/min to allow for maximal future viability of cells.
6. Leaving cells at −80 °C is not acceptable for long-term storage (>1 month) and will lead to decreased cell viability.
7. For 386- and 1536-well plate formats, changing media is not feasible, so cells should be plated sparsely enough that they do not deplete media before the plates are read.
8. NPC proliferation consistently decreases around passage 18–20. Bank a large number of early passage (e.g., P6) NPCs to ensure enough cells to carry out screen.
9. In the authors' experience, NPCs plated at this density are viable for at least 96 h, without changing media.
10. Z' and minimum Z value used to determine hits need be individualized for each assay. Positive and negative controls should be chosen carefully to maximize your Z' value.

Acknowledgments

This work was supported by grants from the National Institutes of Health (R01MH078972 to XZ, U54HD090256to the Waisman Center), John Merck Fund (to XZ and AB), Jenni and Kyle Professorship (to XZ), and a Rath Graduate Fellowship to JH.

References

1. Debnath A, Parsonage D, Andrade RM et al (2012) A high-throughput drug screen for Entamoeba histolytica identifies a new lead and target. Nat Med 18:956–960
2. Gupta PB, Onder TT, Jiang G et al (2009) Identification of selective inhibitors of Cancer stem cells by high-throughput screening. Cell 138:645–659
3. Ma T, Thiagarajah JR, Yang H et al (2002) Thiazolidinone CFTR inhibitor identified by high-throughput screening blocks cholera toxin–induced intestinal fluid secretion. J Clin Invest 110:1651–1658
4. Li M, Zhao H, Ananiev GE et al (2017) Establishment of reporter lines for detecting fragile X mental retardation (*FMR1*) gene reactivation in human neural cells: *FMR1* reporter human iPSC line. Stem Cells 35:158–169
5. Chambers SM, Fasano CA, Papapetrou EP et al (2009) Highly efficient neural conversion of human ES and iPS cells by dual inhibition of SMAD signaling. Nat Biotechnol 27:275–280

Chapter 8

Modeling FXS: Human Pluripotent Stem Cells and In Vitro Neural Differentiation

Liron Kuznitsov-Yanovsky, Yoav Mayshar, and Dalit Ben-Yosef

Abstract

In fragile X syndrome (FXS) embryos FMRP is widely expressed during early stages of embryogenesis however it is inactivated by the end of the first trimester. In the same manner, human embryonic stem cell (hESC) lines from FXS blastocysts, bearing the full CGG expansion mutation, express FMRP in their pluripotent stage and in neurons derived following in vitro differentiation, *FMR1* is completely silenced. Therefore, in vitro neural differentiation of FX-hESC lines serves as a uniquely valuable model system to study the developmental mechanisms underlying FXS, together with the proper differentiation protocol to mimic the neurodevelopmental process occurs in vivo.

Key words Pluripotent human embryonic stem cells, In vitro neural differentiation, Dual-SMAD inhibition

1 Introduction

Several in vivo and in vitro models are currently being used to investigate FX pathologies. *FMR1* knockout (KO) models have been previously generated, mainly in mice [1, 2] but also in zebrafish and drosophila [3, 4]. However, there are obviously many substantial differences both in the gross anatomical level and in the fine structure between the human brain, and that of rodent animal models. In addition, since the inactivation of *FMR1* occurs only during development of the human FX fetus, KO models which do not express *FMR1* even at an early stage of development may serve as a tool for studying the molecular function of FMRP, but they lack the ability of simulating the progression of the disease. The human in vitro models available are post-mortem adult neurons or neural precursor cells (NPCs), NPCs extracted from aborted fetuses [5–8], and induced pluripotent stem cells (iPSCs) generated from fibroblasts of FX individuals [9–11]. Significantly, none of these human in vitro models express *FMR1* at early stages of development, similar to the natural human fetus.

Dalit Ben-Yosef and Yoav Mayshar (eds.), *Fragile-X Syndrome: Methods and Protocols*, Methods in Molecular Biology, vol. 1942, https://doi.org/10.1007/978-1-4939-9080-1_8, © Springer Science+Business Media, LLC, part of Springer Nature 2019

Human embryonic stem cells (hESCs) are pluripotent cells derived from the inner cell mass of preimplantation blastocysts. They can grow indefinitely in culture, while keeping their potential to differentiate into all cell types in the human body, thus serving as an important research tool in developmental biology and the studying of genetic disorders, as well as a valuable resource for drug screening and regenerative medicine. In FX fetuses, FMRP is expressed up to 12.5 weeks of pregnancy (seen by chorionic villi samples; [12]), suggesting its functionality during most of the critical period of embryonic brain development. FX-hESCs lines derived from FX affected blastocysts, carry the full natural mutation at the *FMR1* gene, and express *FMR1* in their pluripotent stage [13, 14]. *FMR1* is gradually silenced in male FX-hESCs along with differentiation; similar to the process which occurs in human FX fetuses during pregnancy [12].

Neurons comprise neuronal networks, and the synapses are essential to neuronal function by permitting a neuron to pass an electrical or chemical signal to another neuron. Generation of functional neuronal networks following in vitro neural differentiation of FX-hESCs is critical for better understanding of the pathophysiology underlying FXS [14–16]. While FXS neurons can fire single action potentials (APs), unlike healthy control cells they are unable to discharge trains of APs. In addition, these human FXS neurons contain fewer synaptic vesicles and lack spontaneous synaptic activity [16]. Neural differentiation of FX-iPSCs maintained the DNA methylation status at the *FMR1* locus during differentiation which was correlated with the gene's expression [17]. In addition, differentiated FX-iPSCs showed a slight neurodevelopmental delay and more immature synaptic network, compared to *FRM1* expressing cells. Collectively, neural differentiation of FX-PSCs can serve as a highly relevant system for studying the neurodevelopmental aspects of FXS and for analyzing the molecular mechanisms leading to the functional deficiencies of its neurons.

Using the dual SMAD inhibition protocol neuronal cultures were generated from hESCs, expressing neuronal genes. In this protocol, neural specification to generate neural precursors is induced by the inhibition of both TGF-beta and BMP signaling pathways with small molecules resulting in suppression of mesoendodermal and trophoblast fates, causing the creation of a neuroepithelial cell sheet and directing the differentiation toward neuroectoderm [18–20]. This swift induction is due to the blocking of SMAD signaling transduction by two inhibitors, SB-431542 and dorsomorphin [21–23]. Afterward, hESCs are subjected to neuronal growth factors (BDNF, GDNF, and NT-3) together with other supplementations to induce neuronal specification. Functional neurons are derived within 2–3 months, as evidenced by their ability to fire repetitive action potential and synaptic currents [14]. However, they are somewhat immature compared to primary adult neurons, as determined by the complexity of the neurons' projections, the density of the neuronal network, and the frequency of synaptic currents [15].

Recently, an optimization of this protocol was reported by the addition of combined small molecules; WNT antagonist, inhibitors of FGF and Notch signaling, and MAPK/ERK kinase inhibitor. Inhibition of WNT signaling blocks the formation of neural crest cells and enhances the induction of forebrain precursors [24], inhibition of FGF & Notch signaling, as well as of MAPK/ERK kinase, which is downstream of FGF receptor activation, is required for exiting pluripotency in hPSCs and enhancing overall neuroectodermal differentiation [25, 26]. This protocol had been shown to accelerate, in a more efficient, rapid, and reproducible manner, the generation of functional cortical neurons from hESCs or iPSCs, when over 50% of the cells are Tuj1^{+} within 13 days [27].

2 Materials

2.1 Human PSC Culture

1. Coating medium: DMEM medium, stored at 4 °C.
2. Geltrex™ LDEV-Free Reduced Growth Factor Basement Membrane Matrix. Aliquot and store in −20 °C (*see* **Note 1**).
3. mTeSR™1 medium: 400 ml mTeSR™1 Basal medium and 100 ml mTeSR™1 5× Supplement, 1 ml Primocin (100 μg/ml). Store at 4 °C for a maximum of 2 weeks. Bring to room temperature before usage.
4. ROCK inhibitor: After passage, cells are plated in mTeSR™1 medium supplemented with 5 μM final concentration Y-276321 ROCK inhibitor (ROCKi). Aliquots of 5 mM stock ROCKi are stored at 4 °C for a maximum of 2 weeks.
5. Dissociation reagent: Accutase. Store aliquots at −20 °C, and at 4 °C for a maximum of 2 month.
6. Freezing medium: CryoStem™ Freezing Medium. Store at 4 °C.

2.2 Neural and Neuronal Induction of hPSCs by Dual SMAD Inhibition

1. SB-431542 10 mM stock solution: dissolve 10 mg SB-431542 powder in 2.6 ml DMSO. Store aliquots at −80 °C.
2. Dorsomorphin 5 mM stock solution: dissolve 2 mg dorsomorphin powder in 815.6 μl DMSO. Store aliquots at −80 °C.
3. hES medium: KO-DMEM medium, 20% v/v knockout serum replacement, 1% v/v nonessential amino acids, 1% GlutaMAX, 1% insulin–transferrin–selenium (ITS), 0.1 mM β-mercaptoethanol, 100 μg/ml Primocin, supplemented fresh every day for the first 10 days with 10 μM SB-431542 from a stock of 10 mM in DMSO and 5 μM dorsomorphin from a stock of 5 mM in DMSO. Store at 4 °C for a maximum of 2 weeks.

4. N2B27 medium composed of 1:1 combination of N2 medium and B27 medium. N2 medium is composed of: DMEM/F-12, 1% N2, 1% GlutaMAX, 1% nonessential amino acids, 100 μg/ml Primocin. B27 medium is composed of Neurobasal, 1% B27, 1% GlutaMAX, 100 μg/ml Primocin. From day 12, N2B27 medium is supplemented fresh with a final concentration of 20 ng/ml recombinant Human BDNF from 10 μg/ml stock, a final concentration of 20 ng/ml recombinant Human GDNF from 10 μg/ml stock, a final concentration of 20 ng/ml recombinant Human NT3 from 10 μg/ml stock, 0.2 mM ascorbic acid, 0.5 mM dibutyryl cyclic-AMP (dbcAMP), and 10 μM DAPT.
5. 50 μg/ml poly-L-ornithine solution.
6. Laminin solution: Dissolve 1 ml of 1 mg/ml Laminin in 49 ml of PBS (20 μg/ml stock). Aliquot and freeze at −20 °C. Before use, thaw it slowly on ice.

2.3 Neural Induction of hPSCs by Accelerated Combined Small-Molecule Inhibition

1. KSR medium: KO-DMEM, 15% v/v knockout serum replacement, 1 mM L-glutamine (0.5%), 100 μM MEM nonessential amino acids (1%), 0.1 mM β-mercaptoethanol.
2. N2/B27 medium: DMEM-F12, 1% N2, 1% B27, (0.5%) 1 mM L-glutamine.
3. NB/B27 medium: Neurobasal, 1% B27, (0.5%) 1 mM L-glutamine.

   Compounds supplemented to the above media in the different days (*see* Subheading 3 for details):

   (a) 250 nM LDN193189 from a stock solution of 250 μM in DMSO.

   (b) 10 μM SB431542 from a stock solution of 10 mM in DMSO.

   (c) 5 μM XAV939 from a stock solution of 5 mM in DMSO.

   (d) 1 μM in P1S5D, 8 μM in P8S10D PD0325901 from a stock solution of 1 mM or 8 mM in DMSO, respectively (*see* **Note 8**).

   (e) 5 μM in P1S5D, 10 μM in P8S10D SU5402 from a stock solution of 5 mM or 10 mM in DMSO, respectively (*see* **Note 8**).

   (f) 10 μM DAPT from a stock solution of 10 mM in DMSO.

   (g) 20 ng/ml BDNF from a stock solution of 10 μg/ml in DDW.

   (h) 0.2 mM ascorbic acid from a stock solution of 100 mM in DDW.

   (i) 0.5 mM dbcAMP from a stock solution of 100 mM in DDW.

4. 15 μg/ml polyornithine solution in PBS.
5. 1 μg/ml mouse laminin I solution in PBS.
6. 2 μg/ml fibronectin solution in PBS.

3 Methods

3.1 Human PSCs Culture

1. For the coating of cell culture plates: Thaw Geltrex® Matrix solution on ice, place desired tissue plates in 4 °C. Mix Geltrex® Matrix solution by slowly pipetting up and down; be careful not to introduce air bubbles and dilute 1:100 (e.g., add 60 μl Geltrex® Matrix solution into 6 ml prechilled, 4 °C, DMEM medium, 1% final concentration). Add sufficient diluted Geltrex® Matrix solution to cover the entire growth surface area (e.g., 1 ml for one 6 well). The coated dish is stable for 2 weeks when wrapped with Parafilm® sealing film and stored at 4 °C. Do not allow coated surface to dry out. It is critical to maintain a storage temperature of 4 °C to avoid premature gelling. Incubate coated plates at 37 °C for a minimum of 60 min. At time of use, it is recommended to keep plates at room temperature for 1 h before aspirating. Carefully aspirate the supernatant above the Geltrex® coating and immediately plate cells in pre-equilibrated cell culture medium.
2. To create a confluent hPSC monolayer for neural induction, thaw frozen hPSCs from liquid nitrogen for 1 min in 37 °C water bath. Transfer to a 15 ml tube with 5 ml DMEM. Centrifuge at 300 × *g* for 5 min and aspirate the supernatant. Resuspend the cell pellet in mTeSR™1 supplemented with ROCKi (1:1000 dilutions) and transfer to a Geltrex-coated cell culture and place in the incubator (37 °C, 5% CO_2). The next day, refresh with new mTeSR™1 without ROCKi. Change the medium every other day until the next passaging (*see* **Note 2**).
3. To Passage hPSCs, aspirate the culture medium and wash once with 1× PBS without Ca^{2+} and Mg^{2+}. Dissociate the cells by adding ~300 μl Accutase to coat the well and place in the incubator (37 °C, 5% CO_2) for about 3 min, till colonies detach and become single cells. Add 1 ml DMEM and pipet cells a few times to make a single cell suspension and transfer to a 15 ml tube with 5 ml DMEM. *Optional: add another 1 ml DMEM to wash the well and transfer to the 15 ml tube.* Centrifuge cells at 300 × *g* for 5 min. Aspirate supernatant, briefly tap the tube and resuspend with mTeSR™1 supplemented with ROCKi (1:1000 dilutions), seed onto Geltrex-coated plates in a split-ratio of 1:4 (*see* **Note 3**). The next day, refresh with new mTeSR™1 without ROCKi. Change medium every other day until cells are ~80–90% confluent. Passage is usually every 3–4 days.

4. To freeze hPSCs, dissociate the cells by adding ~300 μl Accutase to coat the well and place in the incubator (37 °C, 5% CO_2) for about 3 min, till colonies detach and become single cells. Add 1 ml DMEM and pipet cells a few times to make a single cell suspension and transfer to a 15 ml tube with 5 ml DMEM. *Optional: add another 1 ml DMEM to wash the well and transfer to the 15 ml tube.* Centrifuge cells at 300 × *g* for 5 min. Aspirate supernatant, briefly tap the tube and resuspend with CryoStem™ Freezing Medium. Aliquot into cryotubes as desired and put the tubes in a freezing container, store at −80 °C for at least 2 h. For long term, store in liquid nitrogen.

3.2 Dual SMAD Inhibition

The dual-SMAD inhibition protocol is adapted from Chambers et al. [19]; and from our experience as described in Telias et al. [16]. An outline of the differentiation scheme is presented in Fig. 1.

1. *Neural induction*: When hPSC cultures are 80–90% confluent (*see* **Note 4**), conduct neural induction by switching the medium to hES medium supplemented with 10 μM SB-431542 and 5 μM Dorsomorphin, defined as **D0** of the differentiation.
2. On day 2 of differentiation, aspirate the hES and add fresh hES with 10 μM SB431542 and 5 μM dorsomorphin.
3. On day 4 of differentiation, aspirate the hES and add a mixture of hES and N2B27 (3:1), with 10 μM SB431542 and 5 μM dorsomorphin.
4. On day 6 of differentiation, aspirate the medium and add a mixture of hES and N2B27 (1:1), with 10 μM SB431542 and 5 μM Dorsomorphin.
5. On day 8 of differentiation, aspirate the medium and add a mixture of hES and N2B27 (1:3), with 10 μM SB431542 and 5 μM Dorsomorphin.

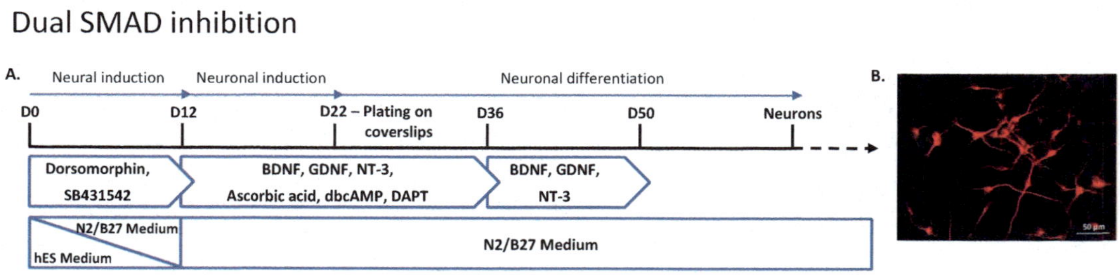

Fig. 1 In vitro differentiation of neurons from human embryonic stem cells by dual SMAD inhibition (**a**) Schematic presentation of the protocol for in vitro neural differentiation using the dual SMAD inhibition. (**b**) Representative images of Hues 13 WT-hESC-derived neurons at day 62 of differentiation, stained positive for MAP2 (red).

6. On day 10 of differentiation, aspirate the medium and add fresh N2B27 with 10 μM SB431542 and 5 μM Dorsomorphin.
7. On day 12 of differentiation, and every 2 days until day 20 (included), aspirate the N2B27 and add fresh N2B27 supplemented with final concentration of 20 ng/ml BDNF, 20 ng/ml GDNF, 20 ng/ml NT-3, 0.2 mM ascorbic acid, 0.5 mM dbcAMP, and 10 μM DAPT.
8. *Neuronal induction*: Prepare 24-well plate with coverslips (*see* **Note 5**):
   (a) On day 20, after placing the coverslips in the 24-wells, add EtOH 70% for 20 min and wash twice with sterile DDW. Add 300 μl cold polyornithine. Leave for 24 h in 37 °C.
   (b) On day 21, aspirate the polyornithine and wash twice with DDW. Add 300 μl of diluted laminin. Seal with Parafilm and place in 37 °C overnight.
9. On day 22, aspirate N2B27 media and add ~300 μl Accutase to coat the well. Place in the incubator (37 °C, 5% CO_2) for about 10 min, till cells detach. Add 1 ml N2B27 and pipet cells a few times to make a single cell suspension and transfer to a 15 ml tube with 5 ml N2B27 without supplements. *Optional: add another 1 ml N2B27 to wash the well and transfer to the 15 ml tube*. Centrifuge cells at 300 × *g* for 5 min. Prepare N2B27 with final concentration of 20 ng/ml BDNF, 20 ng/ml GDNF, 20 ng/ml NT-3, 0.2 mM ascorbic acid, 0.5 mM dbcAMP, and 10 μM DAPT, 1 ml per 24 well. Aspirate supernatant, briefly tap the tube and rinse pellet with ~40 μl for each coverslip that the cells will be seeded on as initial drop-seeding (*see* **Note 6**). Pipet gently ~10 times with a 200 μl-tip. Aspirate laminin from the coverslips and wash it twice with PBS. Place one drop of 40–50 μl containing cells in the center of the coverslip. Incubate for 1 h in the incubator (37 °C, 5% CO_2). After 1 h, add 1 ml of medium (N2B27 + all supplements) to each well, by making it flow carefully through the wall of the well (*see* **Note 7**). Change medium twice a week, aspirate only 0.5 ml and add fresh 0.5 ml.
   (a) For the first 2 weeks use N2B27 with all supplements (as in days 10–20 of the neural induction).
   (b) For weeks 3 and 4 use N2B27 and add only BDNF, GDNF, and NT-3.
   (c) From week 5 and on use N2B27 without any supplement.

3.3 Accelerated Induction of Cortical Neurons

The accelerated protocol is adapted from Qi et al. [27]. An outline of the differentiation scheme is presented in Fig. 2.

1. When hPSC cultures are 80–90% confluent (*see* **Note 4**), conduct neural induction by switching the medium to KSR

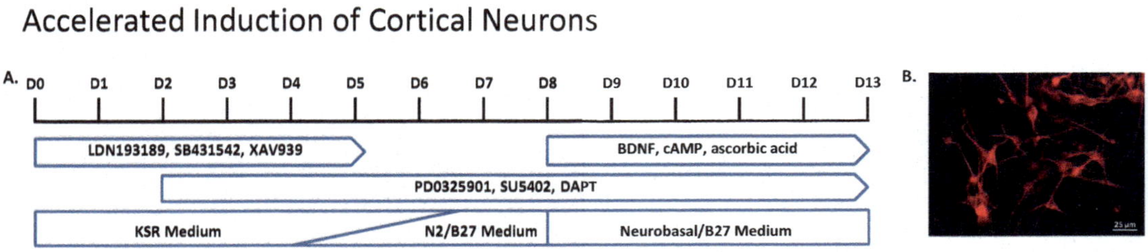

Fig. 2 In vitro differentiation of neurons from human embryonic stem cells by the combined small-molecule accelerated protocol (**a**) Schematic presentation of the protocol for accelerated in vitro neural differentiation using the combined small-molecule accelerated protocol. (**b**) Representative images of Hues 13 WT-hESC-derived neurons at day 13 of differentiation, stained positive for MAP2 (red)

medium supplemented with 250 nM LDN193189, 10 μM SB431542 and 5 μM XAV939, defined as **D0** of the differentiation.

2. On day 1 of differentiation, aspirate the KSR and add fresh KSR with 250 nM LDN193189, 10 μM SB431542, and 5 μM XAV939.
3. On days 2 and 3 of differentiation, aspirate the KSR and add fresh KSR with 250 nM LDN193189, 10 μM SB431542, 5 μM XAV939, 1 μM (in P1S5D) or 8 μM (in P8S10D) PD0325901, 5 μM (in P1S5D) or 10 μM (in P8S10D) SU5402, and 10 μM DAPT (*see* **Note 8**).
4. On days 4 and 5 of differentiation, aspirate the KSR and add a mixture of KSR and N2B27 (3:1) with 250 nM LDN193189, 10 μM SB431542, 5 μM XAV939, 1 μM (in P1S5D) or 8 μM (in P8S10D) PD0325901, 5 μM (in P1S5D) or 10 μM (in P8S10D) SU5402, and 10 μM DAPT.
5. On days 6 and 7 of differentiation, aspirate the medium and add a mixture of KSR and N2B27 (1:3) with 1 μM (in P1S5D) or 8 μM (in P8S10D) PD0325901, 5 μM (in P1S5D) or 10 μM (in P8S10D) SU5402, and 10 μM DAPT.
6. On days 8, 9, 11 and 13 of differentiation, aspirate the medium and add fresh NB/B27 with 1 μM (in P1S5D) or 8 μM (in P8S10D) PD0325901, 5 μM (in P1S5D) or 10 μM (in P8S10D) SU5402, 10 μM DAPT, 20 ng/ml BDNF, 0.5 mM dbcAMP, and 0.2 mM ascorbic acid.
7. *For long-term culture beyond day 13* for the generation of deep and upper layer neurons, differentiate the cells as described above till day 8, and then passage onto polyornithine–laminin–fibronectin-coated dishes. Coat the dishes with polyornithine (15 μg/ml) diluted in PBS for 24 h at 37 °C. Wash with PBS, and further coat the dishes with mouse laminin I (1 μg/ml) and fibronectin (2 μg/ml) diluted in PBS for 12 hrs at 37 °C. Remove laminin and fibronectin immediately before use.

8. Dissociate day 8 cells with Accutase at 37 °C for ~20 min. Wash the cells and plate onto polyornithine–laminin–fibronectin-coated dishes at 150,000 cells/cm^2 (for P1S5D protocol) or 300,000 cells/cm^2 (for P8S10D protocol), respectively (*see* **Note 9**), in NB/B27 + BDNF + dbcAMP + ascorbic acid (*see* **Note 10**).
9. Change medium (NB/B27 + BDNF + dbcAMP + ascorbic acid) every 3–4 days, and 1 μg/ml laminin can be added weekly for better attachment of neurons.

4 Notes

1. Geltrex should be slowly thawed overnight in an ice-bucket in 4 °C. Aliquots of 60 μl are distributed quickly the next day and kept in −20 °C.
2. For each 6 well use 2 ml of medium, 1 ml for one 12 well and 0.5 ml for one 24 well, and refresh every other day. Cells can also be left for the weekend with 3 ml of medium for one 6 well, 1.5 ml for one 12 well, and 1 ml for one 24 well.
3. We found that passaging ratio of 1:4 is ideal for daily maintenance of our cell culture. However, this dilution can vary between lines and therefore should be adapted accordingly (e.g., higher ratio in order to delay confluence or lower ratio in order to precede confluence).
4. Monolayer neural differentiation protocols require a high cell density for generation of neural precursor cells with high efficiencies. Hence, for best results, differentiation should be executed when cells are at least 80% confluence. In addition, it is recommended to start differentiation at least 2 days after passaging and *not* the day after passage when the ROCKi is present in the medium, but refresh medium the day after passaging and execute the differentiation the day after that.
5. Coverslips for culturing neurons can also be coated with Geltrex™. In addition, if differentiation is conducted for assays which do not require coverslips (e.g., RNA extraction), at day 22 cells can be replated on regular 24-well plates coated with Geltrex. In this case, instead of drop-seeding, plate the cells regularly in supplemented medium (since there is no need to center the cells on a coverslip and the cells can grow on the entire surface of the well).
6. We use seeding density of ~1.0×10^5 cells/cm^2 for WT-cells. However, seeding density varies between the lines and should be adapted accordingly.
7. Before drop-seeding, make sure the coverslips are well attached to the well by pressing with a 200 μl-tip. After adding the 1 ml

medium on the outer sides of the coverslip, press the coverslip again to attach. Repeat this every time medium is refreshed and the coverslip has detached.

8. There are two optional protocols in which different concentrations of two small molecules are used, termed P1S5D protocol and P8S10D protocol: 1 μM PD0325901 and 5 μM SU5402 vs. 8 μM PD0325901 and 10 μM SU5402, respectively. Both methods produce mature neuron, however while P1S5D protocol results in a higher yield of live cells, P8S10D protocol results in a more rapid neuronal maturation together with lower yield of live cells. In our hands, P8S10D protocol is too aggressive for some of the cell lines, and thus protocol should be adapted individually for each cell line.
9. This is the recommended seeding density for the long term culture of neurons; however it should be tested individually for each cell line.
10. While it is very much possible to produce mature electrophysiologically active neurons using this protocol, it can also be improved by treating the cells from day 8 onward with NB/B27 + BDNF + dbcAMP + ascorbic acid together with the addition of DAPT (10 μM) or with the addition of DAPT (10 μM) with SU5402 (5 μM), PD0325901 (1 μM) and CHIR99021 (3 μM). The WNT agonist CHIR99021 can be included for this final differentiation step since it has a strong prosurvival effect. In addition, it has been previously shown that canonical WNT signaling activation promotes neuronal differentiation including axonal outgrowth and synapse formation [28, 29].

References

1. Levenga J, de Vrij FM, Buijsen RA, Li T, Nieuwenhuizen IM, Pop A, Oostra BA, Willemsen R (2011) Subregion-specific dendritic spine abnormalities in the hippocampus of Fmr1 KO mice. Neurobiol Learn Mem 95(4):467–472. https://doi.org/10.1016/j.nlm.2011.02.009
2. Nimchinsky EA, Oberlander AM, Svoboda K (2001) Abnormal development of dendritic spines in FMR1 knock-out mice. J Neurosci 21(14):5139–5146
3. Gatto CL, Broadie K (2008) Temporal requirements of the fragile X mental retardation protein in the regulation of synaptic structure. Development 135(15):2637–2648. https://doi.org/10.1242/dev.022244
4. Ng MC, Yang YL, Lu KT (2013) Behavioral and synaptic circuit features in a zebrafish model of fragile X syndrome. PLoS One 8(3): e51456. https://doi.org/10.1371/journal.pone.0051456
5. Irwin SA, Patel B, Idupulapati M, Harris JB, Crisostomo RA, Larsen BP, Kooy F, Willems PJ, Cras P, Kozlowski PB, Swain RA, Weiler IJ, Greenough WT (2001) Abnormal dendritic spine characteristics in the temporal and visual cortices of patients with fragile-X syndrome: a quantitative examination. Am J Med Genet 98(2):161–167
6. Castren M, Tervonen T, Karkkainen V, Heinonen S, Castren E, Larsson K, Bakker CE, Oostra BA, Akerman K (2005) Altered differentiation of neural stem cells in fragile X syndrome. Proc Natl Acad Sci U S A 102(49):17834–17839. https://doi.org/10.1073/pnas.0508995102
7. Schwartz PH, Tassone F, Greco CM, Nethercott HE, Ziaeian B, Hagerman RJ, Hagerman

PJ (2005) Neural progenitor cells from an adult patient with fragile X syndrome. BMC Med Genet 6:2. https://doi.org/10.1186/1471-2350-6-2

8. Bhattacharyya A, McMillan E, Wallace K, Tubon TC Jr, Capowski EE, Svendsen CN (2008) Normal neurogenesis but abnormal gene expression in human fragile X cortical progenitor cells. Stem Cells Dev 17 (1):107–117. https://doi.org/10.1089/scd.2007.0073
9. Sheridan SD, Theriault KM, Reis SA, Zhou F, Madison JM, Daheron L, Loring JF, Haggarty SJ (2011) Epigenetic characterization of the FMR1 gene and aberrant neurodevelopment in human induced pluripotent stem cell models of fragile X syndrome. PLoS One 6(10): e26203. https://doi.org/10.1371/journal.pone.0026203
10. Urbach A, Bar-Nur O, Daley GQ, Benvenisty N (2010) Differential modeling of fragile X syndrome by human embryonic stem cells and induced pluripotent stem cells. Cell Stem Cell 6(5):407–411. https://doi.org/10.1016/j.stem.2010.04.005
11. Halevy T, Czech C, Benvenisty N (2015) Molecular mechanisms regulating the defects in fragile X syndrome neurons derived from human pluripotent stem cells. Stem Cell Reports 4(1):37–46. https://doi.org/10.1016/j.stemcr.2014.10.015
12. Willemsen R, Bontekoe CJ, Severijnen LA, Oostra BA (2002) Timing of the absence of FMR1 expression in full mutation chorionic villi. Hum Genet 110(6):601–605. https://doi.org/10.1007/s00439-002-0723-5
13. Eiges R, Urbach A, Malcov M, Frumkin T, Schwartz T, Amit A, Yaron Y, Eden A, Yanuka O, Benvenisty N, Ben-Yosef D (2007) Developmental study of fragile X syndrome using human embryonic stem cells derived from preimplantation genetically diagnosed embryos. Cell Stem Cell 1(5):568–577. https://doi.org/10.1016/j.stem.2007.09.001
14. Telias M, Segal M, Ben-Yosef D (2013) Neural differentiation of fragile X human embryonic stem cells reveals abnormal patterns of development despite successful neurogenesis. Dev Biol 374(1):32–45. https://doi.org/10.1016/j.ydbio.2012.11.031
15. Telias M, Segal M, Ben-Yosef D (2014) Electrical maturation of neurons derived from human embryonic stem cells. F1000Res 3:196. https://doi.org/10.12688/f1000research.4943.2
16. Telias M, Kuznitsov-Yanovsky L, Segal M, Ben-Yosef D (2015) Functional deficiencies in fragile X neurons derived from human embryonic stem cells. J Neurosci 35 (46):15295–15306. https://doi.org/10.1523/JNEUROSCI.0317-15.2015
17. Boland MJ, Nazor KL, Tran HT, Szucs A, Lynch CL, Paredes R, Tassone F, Sanna PP, Hagerman RJ, Loring JF (2017) Molecular analyses of neurogenic defects in a human pluripotent stem cell model of fragile X syndrome. Brain 140(3):582–598. https://doi.org/10.1093/brain/aww357
18. Smith JR, Vallier L, Lupo G, Alexander M, Harris WA, Pedersen RA (2008) Inhibition of activin/nodal signaling promotes specification of human embryonic stem cells into neuroectoderm. Dev Biol 313(1):107–117. https://doi.org/10.1016/j.ydbio.2007.10.003
19. Chambers SM, Fasano CA, Papapetrou EP, Tomishima M, Sadelain M, Studer L (2009) Highly efficient neural conversion of human ES and iPS cells by dual inhibition of SMAD signaling. Nat Biotechnol 27(3):275–280. https://doi.org/10.1038/nbt.1529
20. Shi Y, Kirwan P, Smith J, Robinson HP, Livesey FJ (2012) Human cerebral cortex development from pluripotent stem cells to functional excitatory synapses. Nat Neurosci 15(3):477–486. https://doi.org/10.1038/nn.3041
21. Inman GJ, Nicolas FJ, Callahan JF, Harling JD, Gaster LM, Reith AD, Laping NJ, Hill CS (2002) SB-431542 is a potent and specific inhibitor of transforming growth factor-beta superfamily type I activin receptor-like kinase (ALK) receptors ALK4, ALK5, and ALK7. Mol Pharmacol 62(1):65–74
22. Boergermann JH, Kopf J, Yu PB, Knaus P (2010) Dorsomorphin and LDN-193189 inhibit BMP-mediated Smad, p38 and Akt signalling in C2C12 cells. Int J Biochem Cell Biol 42(11):1802–1807. https://doi.org/10.1016/j.biocel.2010.07.018
23. Lippmann ES, Estevez-Silva MC, Ashton RS (2014) Defined human pluripotent stem cell culture enables highly efficient neuroepithelium derivation without small molecule inhibitors. Stem Cells 32(4):1032–1042. https://doi.org/10.1002/stem.1622
24. Maroof AM, Keros S, Tyson JA, Ying SW, Ganat YM, Merkle FT, Liu B, Goulburn A, Stanley EG, Elefanty AG, Widmer HR, Eggan K, Goldstein PA, Anderson SA, Studer L (2013) Directed differentiation and functional maturation of cortical interneurons from human embryonic stem cells. Cell Stem Cell 12(5):559–572. https://doi.org/10.1016/j.stem.2013.04.008
25. Lanner F, Rossant J (2010) The role of FGF/Erk signaling in pluripotent cells.

Development 137(20):3351–3360. https://doi.org/10.1242/dev.050146

26. Greber B, Coulon P, Zhang M, Moritz S, Frank S, Muller-Molina AJ, Arauzo-Bravo MJ, Han DW, Pape HC, Scholer HR (2011) FGF signalling inhibits neural induction in human embryonic stem cells. EMBO J 30 (24):4874–4884. https://doi.org/10.1038/emboj.2011.407
27. Qi Y, Zhang XJ, Renier N, Wu Z, Atkin T, Sun Z, Ozair MZ, Tchieu J, Zimmer B, Fattahi F, Ganat Y, Azevedo R, Zeltner N, Brivanlou AH, Karayiorgou M, Gogos J, Tomishima M, Tessier-Lavigne M, Shi SH, Studer L (2017) Combined small-molecule inhibition accelerates the derivation of functional cortical neurons from human pluripotent stem cells. Nat Biotechnol 35 (2):154–163. https://doi.org/10.1038/nbt.3777
28. Lie DC, Colamarino SA, Song HJ, Desire L, Mira H, Consiglio A, Lein ES, Jessberger S, Lansford H, Dearie AR, Gage FH (2005) Wnt signalling regulates adult hippocampal neurogenesis. Nature 437(7063):1370–1375. https://doi.org/10.1038/nature04108
29. Salinas PC (2012) Wnt signaling in the vertebrate central nervous system: from axon guidance to synaptic function. Cold Spring Harb Perspect Biol 4(2). https://doi.org/10.1101/cshperspect.a008003

Chapter 9

Induced Neurons for the Study of Neurodegenerative and Neurodevelopmental Disorders

Evelyn J. Sauter, Lisa K. Kutsche, Simon D. Klapper, and Volker Busskamp

Abstract

Patient-derived or genomically modified human induced pluripotent stem cells (iPSCs) offer the opportunity to study neurodevelopmental and neurodegenerative disorders. Overexpression of certain neurogenic transcription factors (TFs) in iPSCs can induce efficient differentiation into homogeneous populations of the disease-relevant neuronal cell types. Here we provide protocols for genomic manipulations of iPSCs by CRISPR/Cas9. We also introduce two methods, based on lentiviral delivery and the piggyBac transposon system, to stably integrate neurogenic TFs into human iPSCs. Furthermore, we describe the TF-mediated neuronal differentiation and maturation in combination with astrocyte cocultures.

Key words Human induced pluripotent stem cells, Nucleofection, PiggyBac transposon, Lentiviral transduction, CRISPR/Cas9, Transcription factor-mediated neuronal differentiation, Astrocyte coculture

1 Introduction

Induced pluripotent stem cells (iPSCs) enable studying neurodevelopmental and neurodegenerative diseases such as autism spectrum disorders including fragile X syndrome and Rett syndrome, amyotrophic lateral sclerosis, Alzheimer's disease, Parkinson's disease, Huntington's disease, or spinal muscular atrophy [1]. Human iPSC lines are generated by reprogramming of fibroblasts, hair, or blood samples [2], which are either directly donated by patients with a disease-relevant phenotype and a known genotype or disease-causing mutations can be introduced into the genome of the iPSCs by genomic modifications such as CRISPR/Cas9 [3]. To study the effect of the mutations on the cellular level, iPSCs can be differentiated into the disease-relevant neuronal subtypes. Conventional differentiation protocols rely on the addition of specific soluble growth factors and compounds to the culturing media. These factors trigger intracellular signaling pathways affecting

Dalit Ben-Yosef and Yoav Mayshar (eds.), *Fragile-X Syndrome: Methods and Protocols*, Methods in Molecular Biology, vol. 1942, https://doi.org/10.1007/978-1-4939-9080-1_9, © The Author(s) 2019

transcription factors (TFs), which in turn induce neuronal differentiation by changing gene expression levels and triggering gene regulatory networks. However, these protocols can be very delicate and time-consuming, lasting from several weeks to months, and yield a heterogeneous mixture of different neuronal subtypes at different developmental stages and glia cells. The forced expression of certain neurogenic TFs in human iPSCs shortcuts neuronal differentiation resulting in rapid neurogenesis that yields highly homogeneous populations of neurons [4–7]. Here we describe the culturing of a robust inducible-neuronal iPSC line as well as different methods to introduce neurogenic TFs and genomic modifications into human iPSCs and how to differentiate those iPSCs into mature neurons.

Neurogenic TFs under the control of a doxycycline-inducible promoter can be stably integrated in the genome of iPSCs either by lentiviral delivery [8] or via the piggyBac transposon system [9]. While lentiviruses have a high efficiency in delivering transgenes, the preparation of viral particles is laborious, time-consuming and requires biosafety level 2. In contrast, the piggyBac transposon system offers a nonviral alternative to efficiently cut and paste transgenes into the genome. The production of plasmids is faster and cheaper and the piggyBac system requires only standard laboratory biosafety levels. For genome editing of human iPSCs with great precision, the CRISPR/Cas9 technology is the method of choice since it is easy-to-use, efficient, and cost-effective. Genomically modified iPSCs can be differentiated into neurons by doxycycline-induced overexpression of TFs and maturation is achieved by astrocyte coculture.

2 Materials

2.1 Human iPSC Culture

1. Human iPSC line with or without genomic modifications (e.g., PGP1 cells (Personal Genome Project iPS cell line, derived from Participant #1 (PGP1, hu43860C)), can be obtained from Coriell #GM23338, the matching primary fibroblast line is #GM23248) or iNGN cells (modified from PGP1, contains the neurogenic TFs Neurogenin-1 and Neurogenin-2 under the control of the doxycycline-inducible promoter. This cell line is part of the ENCODE catalogue (https://www.encodeproject.org) #ENCBS369AAA [4]).
2. Coating medium: DMEM medium, 1% penicillin–streptomycin. Store at 4 °C.
3. Matrigel hESC-qualified matrix (Corning). Store aliquots at −20 °C (*see* **Note 1**).
4. mTeSR™1 medium: 400 ml mTeSR™1 Basal medium (Stemcell Technologies), 100 ml mTeSR™1 5× Supplement

(Stemcell Technologies), 5 ml penicillin–streptomycin, sterile-filter (0.45 μm). Store at 4 °C for a maximum of 2 weeks. Do not prewarm before usage.

5. mTeSR™1 medium with ROCK inhibitor (ROCKi): add ROCK inhibitor to mTeSR™1 medium (3.3 μg/ml final concentration). Store at 4 °C for a maximum of 2 weeks.
6. Dissociation reagent: TrypLE Express (Thermo Fisher Scientific). Store at room temperature.
7. Freezing medium: mFreSR™ (Stemcell Technologies). Store aliquots at −20 °C.
8. 1× PBS pH 7.2 without calcium and magnesium. Store at room temperature.

2.2 Nucleofection of PiggyBac Plasmids

1. 4D-Nucleofector™ System: 4D-Nucleofector™ Core Unit and 4D-Nucleofector™ X-Unit (Lonza).
2. P3 Primary Cell 4D-Nucleofector™ X Kit: Containing the Nucleofector™ Solution, Supplement and 100 μl Cuvettes (Lonza). Store the Nucleofector™ Solution and the Supplement at 4 °C.
3. PiggyBac vector containing the gene of interest under the control of a doxycycline-inducible promoter, such as Addgene plasmid #104454 (*see* **Note 2** and Fig. 2a). Store at −20 °C.
4. Transposase vector, such as System Biosciences #PB210PA-1. Store at −20 °C.
5. Antibiotic: If you would like to select the cells for the integrated piggyBac construct, use the appropriate antibiotic (e.g., blasticidin or puromycin). Store aliquots at −20 °C. After thawing store at 4 °C, protected from light.
6. PiggyBac copy number kit (System Biosciences #PBC100A-1) including UCR1 primer mix, PBcopy primer mix, and cell lysis buffer. Store at 4 °C.
7. Real time PCR master mix, such as Power SYBR® Green PCR Master Mix (Thermo Fisher Scientific). Store at 4 °C.
8. Real time PCR system, such as StepOnePlus™ Real-Time PCR System (Thermo Fisher Scientific).

2.3 Lentivirus Production and Transduction

1. A highly transfectable cell line, such as 293T/17 cells (a gift from Didier Trono; ATCC® #CRL-11268).
2. DMEM with 10% FBS: DMEM medium, 10% FBS, 1% penicillin–streptomycin. Store at 4 °C.
3. DMEM w/o FBS: DMEM medium, 1% penicillin–streptomycin. Store at 4 °C.
4. 1 mg/ml PEI solution (pH 7.1): adjust the pH with 0.1 N NaOH, sterile-filter (0.22 μm), aliquot, and store at −20 °C. After thawing, working aliquots can be stored at 4 °C.

5. Lentiviral vector containing the gene of interest under a doxycycline-inducible promoter (e.g., pLV_TRET_Ngn2-2A-Ngn1 (Addgene plasmid #61471) [4] and pLV_hEF1a_rtTA3 (Addgene plasmid #61472) [4] or pLIX403 (Addgene plasmid #41395)) (*see* **Note 3** and Fig. 3a, b). Store at −20 °C.
6. Viral packaging plasmid psPAX2 (a gift from Didier Trono, Addgene plasmid #12260). Store at −20 °C.
7. Viral envelope plasmid pMD2G (a gift from Didier Trono, Addgene plasmid #12259). Store at −20 °C.
8. 50% PEG 6000 solution. Store at 4 °C.
9. 4 M NaCl solution. Store at 4 °C.
10. PBS pH 7.2 without calcium and magnesium. Store at room temperature.
11. Lenti-X™ GoStix™ (Clontech).
12. Antibiotic: If you would like to select the cells for the integrated lentiviral construct, use the appropriate antibiotic (such as blasticidin or puromycin). Store aliquots at −20 °C, after thawing store at 4 °C, protected from light.
13. DNA extraction kit (e.g., DNeasy® Blood and Tissue Kit (Qiagen)).
14. Albumin plasmid pAlbumin (a gift from Didier Trono, Addgene plasmid #22037). Store at −20 °C.
15. TaqMan® PCR master mix, such as TaqMan® Universal PCR Master Mix (Thermo Fisher Scientific). Store at 4 °C.
16. TaqMan® primer and probes for WPRE and albumin detection (*see* Table 1). Dilute in ddH_2O to a concentration of 10 μM and store at −20 °C.
17. Real time PCR system, such as StepOnePlus™Real-Time PCR System (Thermo Fisher Scientific).

Table 1
TaqMan® primer and probes [8]

Primer	Sequence	Fluorophore
WPRE_forward	GGCACTGACAATTCCGTGGT	
WPRE_reverse	AGGGACGTAGCAGAAGGACG	
WPRE_probe	ACGTCCTTTCCATGGCTGCTCGC	FAM-BHQ
Alb_forward	GCTGTCATCTCTTGTGGGCTGT	
Alb_reverse	ACTCATGGGAGCTGCTGGTTC	
Alb_probe	CCTGTCATGCCCACACAAATCTCTCC	FAM-BHQ

2.4 Genome Editing with CRISPR/Cas9

1. Cas9-sgRNA construct, such as pSpCas9(BB)-2A-Puro (PX459) V2.0 (Addgene plasmid #62988) or pSpCas9(BB)-2A-GFP (PX458) (Addgene plasmid #48138), which is expressing both sgRNA together with the gRNA scaffold as well as the staphylococcus pyogenes Cas9 [10]. Store at −20 °C.
2. 10× T4 Ligation Buffer (New England Biolabs). Store at −20 °C.
3. T4 Polynucleotide Kinase (New England Biolabs). Store at −20 °C.
4. BbsI restriction enzyme (10 U/μl) (Thermo Fisher Scientific). Store at −20 °C.
5. Buffer G (Thermo Fisher Scientific). Store at −20 °C.
6. Calf Intestinal Alkaline Phosphatase (CIP) (New England Biolabs). Store at −20 °C.
7. Electrophoresis gel and chamber.
8. Gel extraction kit, such as QIAquick® Gel Extraction Kit (Qiagen).
9. Ligation kit, such as Mighty Mix ligation kit (Clontech). Store at −20 °C.
10. Chemically competent bacteria (e.g., Stbl3). Store at −80 °C.
11. S.O.C. medium. Store at 4 °C.
12. LB-Antibiotics plates with 100 μg/ml ampicillin. Store at 4 °C.
13. Miniprep kit, such as QIAprep® Spin Miniprep Kit (Qiagen).
14. Sequencing primer, such as 5-′-TTTCTTGGGTAGTTTGCAGTTTT-3′. Dilute in ddH_2O to a concentration of 10 μM and store at −20 °C.
15. 4D-Nucleofector™ System (*see* Subheading 2.2).

2.5 Doxycycline-Induced Differentiation

1. Poly-L-lysine (PLL) solution: Dilute PLL hydrobromide in ddH_2O to a stock concentration of 1 mg/ml. Store at 4 °C.
2. Laminin solution: 1 mg/ml stock. Store aliquots at −20 °C.
3. 1× PBS with calcium and magnesium. Store at 4 °C.
4. Doxycycline solution: dissolve 10 mg doxycycline hyclate powder in 20 ml PBS (0.5 mg/ml = 1000×), sterile-filter (0.22 μm). Store aliquots at −20 °C; after thawing store at 4 °C, protected from light.
5. Differentiation medium: mTeSR™1 medium supplemented with 0.5 μg/ml doxycycline. Store at 4 °C for a maximum of 2 weeks.
6. Maturation medium: 10 ml BrainPhys™ Neuronal Medium (Stemcell Technologies) supplemented with 200 μl NeuroCult™ SM1 Neuronal Supplement (Stemcell Technologies),

100 μl N2 Supplement-A (Stemcell Technologies), 20 μl of 10 μg/ml recombinant Human BDNF to a final concentration of 20 ng/ml (Peprotech), 20 μl of 10 μg/ml recombinant Human GDNF to a final concentration of 20 ng/ml (Peprotech), 98 μl of 50 mg/ml dibutyryl cAMP to a final concentration of 1 mM (Sigma), 50 μl of 40 mM ascorbic acid to a final concentration of 200 nM (Sigma), and 100 μl of 100 × penicillin–streptomycin (*see* **Note 4**). Mix thoroughly. Store at 4 °C for a maximum of 2 weeks.

2.6 Coculturing with Astrocytes

1. Rat primary cortical astrocytes (Thermo Fisher Scientific).
2. Astrocyte medium: DMEM +4.5 g/l D-Glucose +1 mM Pyruvate supplemented with N2 Supplement (Thermo Fisher Scientific), 10% OneShot fetal bovine serum (Thermo Fisher Scientific) and 1% penicillin–streptomycin. Store aliquots at −20 °C. After thawing, working aliquots can be stored at 4 °C for a maximum of 2 weeks.
3. Accutase. Store aliquots at −20 °C.
4. 1 M HCl. Store at room temperature.
5. 100% ethanol. Store at room temperature.
6. Low-melting paraffin. Store at room temperature.
7. 1× PBS with calcium and magnesium. Store at 4 °C.
8. Ara-C: dissolve 11 mg cytosine β-D-arabinofuranoside hydrochloride powder in 15 ml ddH_2O (2.5 mM = 500×), sterile-filter (0.22 μm). Store aliquots at −20 °C, after thawing store at 4 °C for several weeks, protected from light.
9. 1% BSA: 8.7 ml BrainPhys™ Neuronal Medium (Stemcell Technologies) supplemented with 128 μl 1 M HEPES and 1.33 μl 7.5% BSA. Prewarm and use immediately.
10. 0.2% BSA: 4 ml BrainPhys™ Neuronal Medium (Stemcell Technologies) supplemented with 59 μl 1 M HEPES and 1 ml 1% BSA from previous step. Prewarm and use immediately.
11. Minimal maturation medium (*see* **Note 5**): 10 ml BrainPhys™ Neuronal Medium (Stemcell Technologies) supplemented with 200 μl NeuroCult™ SM1 Neuronal Supplement (Stemcell Technologies), 100 μl N2 Supplement-A (Stemcell Technologies), 50 μl of 40 mM ascorbic acid (dissolved in ddH_2O) to a final concentration of 200 nM (Sigma) and 100 μl of 100 × penicillin–streptomycin (*see* **Note 4**). Mix thoroughly. Store at 4 °C for a maximum of 2 weeks.

3 Methods

3.1 Human iPSC Culture

1. For the coating of cell culture plates, resuspend one aliquot of Matrigel in the appropriate amount of cold coating medium (*see* **Note 1**). Add the Matrigel solution to the cell culture plates and distribute equally so that the entire well is covered (*see* **Note 6**). Incubate at room temperature for at least 45 min. Use immediately or store at 4 °C for a maximum of 2 weeks. Prior to use, simply aspirate the coating medium and add the cell suspension. No washing step is required.
2. To thaw iPSCs, get the frozen vials from the liquid nitrogen tank and keep on dry ice. Thaw carefully in a 37 °C water bath or alternatively with the ThawSTAR™ Automated Cell Thawing System (BioCision™) until only a small ice cube remains. Transfer the cell solution to a 15 ml Falcon tube and add dropwise 2–3 ml 1× PBS w/o Ca^{2+} and Mg^{2+}. Spin down at 400 × *g* for 4 min and aspirate the supernatant. Resuspend the cell pellet in mTeSR™1 with ROCKi and transfer to a cell culture plate coated with Matrigel and place in the incubator (37 °C, 5% CO_2). After 24 h, wash the cells once with 1× PBS w/o Ca^{2+} and Mg^{2+} and change the medium to mTeSR™1 w/o ROCKi. Change the medium every day until the next passaging (*see* **Note 7**).
3. In order to passage iPSCs, aspirate the culture medium and wash the cells once with 1× PBS w/o Ca^{2+} and Mg^{2+}. Dissociate the cells by adding TrypLE and place in the incubator for approximately 2–3 min. Add 1× PBS w/o Ca^{2+} and Mg^{2+} and pipet up and down to collect all cells. Transfer the cell solution to a 15 ml Falcon tube and spin down at 400 × *g* for 4 min. Aspirate the supernatant and resuspend the cell pellet in mTeSR™1 with ROCKi. Count the cells using Trypan Blue (e.g., with the Countess™ II FL Automated Cell Counter or hemocytometer) and seed the appropriate number of cells in Matrigel- or poly-L-lysine + laminin-coated cell culture plates (*see* **Note 8**). Mix well and place in the incubator (37 °C, 5% CO_2). After 24 h, wash the cells once with 1× PBS w/o Ca^{2+} and Mg^{2+} and change the medium to mTeSR™1 w/o ROCKi. Change the medium every day until next passaging (*see* **Note 7** and Fig. 1). It is recommended to check the iPSCs regularly for mycoplasma contamination (*see* **Note 9**).
4. To freeze iPSCs, dissociate the cells with TrypLE and collect in 1× PBS w/o Ca^{2+} and Mg^{2+}, spin down and resuspend the pellet in mFreSR™ medium. If necessary, count the cells and aliquot the appropriate amount into cryotubes (*see* **Note 10**). Put the tubes in a freezing container and store at −80 °C for at least 2 h. Subsequently, store in liquid nitrogen.

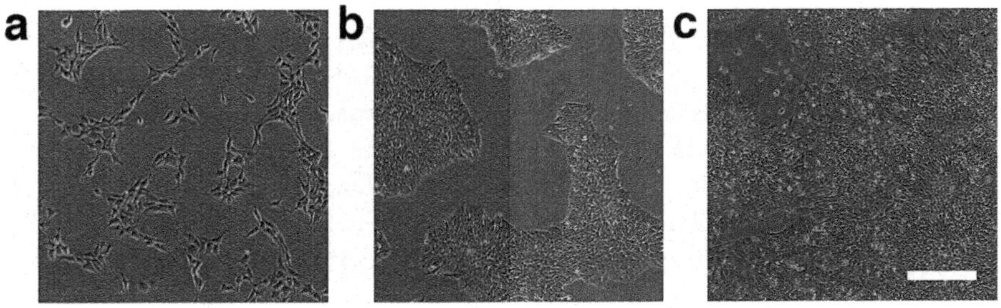

Fig. 1 Representative images of human iPSCs [4] grown on Matrigel-coated cell culture plates. (**a**) iPSCs 1 day after passaging in mTeSR™1 with ROCKi. (**b**) iPSC colonies in mTeSR™1 w/o ROCKi. (**c**) Confluent iPSC colonies. Scale bar represents 200 μm

3.2 Nucleofection of iPSCs

1. In order to electroporate piggyBac and transposase vectors into iPSCs in suspension, use the X-Unit of the 4D-Nucleofector™ System in combination with the P3 Primary Cell 4D-Nucleofector™ X Kit according to the manufacturer's guidelines.
2. First of all, prepare the DNA, the Nucleofector™ solution and the cell culture plates. For a nucleofection reaction in 100 μl cuvettes, mix 10 μg piggyBac vector and 2.5 μg transposase vector in less than 10 μl volume (maximum 10% of the final sample volume) in a 1.5 ml tube. In a separate tube, mix 82 μl Nucleofector™ solution with 18 μl supplement per nucleofection reaction and bring to room temperature. Prepare Matrigel-coated cell culture plates with the desired volume of mTeSR™1 medium with ROCKi and prewarm in the incubator (*see* **Note 11**).
3. Switch on the X-Unit of the 4D-Nucleofector™ System and choose the cell-type specific program for the human embryonic stem cell line H9, the cuvette size, P3 primary solution and the pulse CB-156 or CB-150 (*see* **Note 12**).
4. Dissociate the cells to be nucleofected using TrypLE, centrifuge (400 × *g*, 4 min) and resuspend in mTeSR™1 with ROCKi. Determine the cell number, transfer 800,000 cells for each nucleofection into a 1.5 ml tube and centrifuge (400 × *g*, 4 min). Aspirate the supernatant and resuspend the cells in 100 μl room temperature Nucleofector™ solution with supplement, mix with the DNA and transfer into an electroporation cuvette and close the lid. Avoid air bubbles while pipetting. Gently tap the cuvette to make sure that the sample covers the bottom.
5. Quickly put the cuvette(s) into the Nucleofector™ and press the start button to apply the pulse CB-156 or CB-150. Immediately after, carefully remove the samples, add mTeSR™1 with ROCKi into the cuvette, mix by gently pipetting up and down

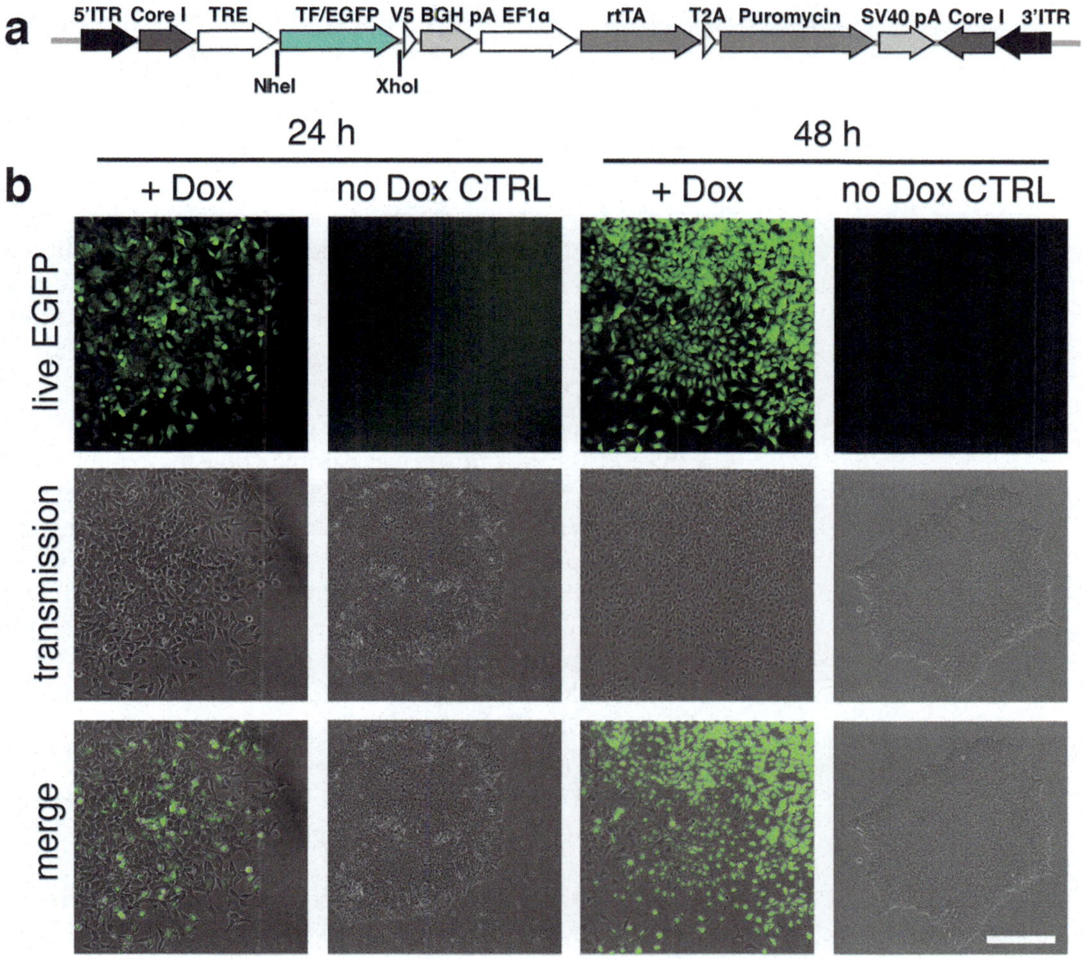

Fig. 2 Nucleofection of iPSCs with the piggyBac plasmid. (**a**) Schematic representation of the piggyBac plasmid containing the 5′ and 3′ inverted terminal repeats (ITR), core insulator (Core I), the doxycycline-inducible TRE promoter driving the expression of a transcription factor (TF) or in our example of EGFP which can be excised be the restriction enzymes NheI and XhoI and replaced by a TF of interest, followed by a V5 tag and a bGH poly A signal. Furthermore, the plasmid contains an EF1α promoter driving the expression of the doxycycline-sensitive transactivator rtTA followed by a T2A signal and a puromycin resistance gene. (**b**) Representative images of iPSCs nucleofected with the plasmid depicted in (**a**) 24 and 48 h after doxycycline (Dox) induction and respective controls without doxycycline (no Dox CTRL). Scale bar represents 200 μm

two to three times and transfer the complete solution onto a Matrigel-coated plate with prewarmed medium and place in the incubator (*see* **Note 13**).

6. The next day, wash the cells with 1× PBS w/o Ca^{2+} and Mg^{2+} and change the medium to mTeSR™1 w/o ROCKi. Change the medium every day until next passaging (*see* Fig. 2b). Starting 48 h after nucleofection, select the cells with an integrated construct with the appropriate antibiotic (*see* **Note 14**).

7. In order to determine the number of the integrated piggyBac constructs, use the piggyBac copy number kit from System Biosciences (*see* **Note 15**). To prepare genomic DNA, seed the cells in a 12-well plate (*see* **Note 16**). When confluent, wash once with 1× PBS w/o Ca^{2+} and Mg^{2+} and add 250 μl lysis buffer to each well. Freeze the cells at −80 °C and thaw the plate at room temperature to ensure complete cellular lysis. Detach the cells by pipetting up and down, transfer the lysates to 1.5 ml tubes and heat them at 95 °C for 2 min. Centrifuge at 17,000 × *g* for 2 min and transfer the supernatant to a new 1.5 ml tube. The lysates should be placed on ice if used immediately or stored at −20 °C.
8. Prepare two master mixes of 4.75 μl ddH_2O, 6.25 μl SYBR® Green, and 0.5 μl primers per sample (one master mix with UCR1 primers for genomic DNA detection and one with PBcopy primers for piggyBac detection). Aliquot 12 μl master mix per well of a 96-well plate and add 0.5 μl lysate (≤500 ng DNA). Seal the plate, carefully mix by vortexing and briefly spin down. Run the qPCR with the following program: 2 min at 50 °C, 10 min at 95 °C, 40 cycles of 95 °C for 15 s and 60 °C for 1 min, followed by 15 s at 95 °C, 15 s at 60 °C, and 15 s at 95 °C (*see* **Note 17**).
9. Calculate the copy number as follows [11]: $\Delta\Delta C_t = 2^{(\text{average PBcopy Ct–average UCR1 } C_t)}$, divide the $\Delta\Delta C_t$ by 2 as there are two copies of the UCR1 sequence per genome.

3.3 Lentivirus Production and Transduction

1. For the production and transduction of lentiviruses, titration and copy number determination, we follow the protocol from the Trono lab [8].
2. One day prior to transfection, seed 8,000,000,293T/17 cells in a 10 cm culture dish. The next day, replace the culture medium with 4 ml fresh DMEM with 10% FBS. The cells are transfected using 45 μg of polyethylenimine (PEI) combined with 15 μg DNA containing the plasmid of interest (*see* Fig. 3a, b), the viral packaging (psPAX2) plasmid, and the viral envelope (pMD2G) plasmid in a 4:2:1 ratio. In detail, mix 45 μl of 1 mg/ml PEI solution with 955 μl DMEM medium w/o FBS in a 1.5 ml tube. In a separate tube, mix 2.1 μg pMD2G, 4.2 μg psPAX2, and 8.4 μg vector of interest with 1 ml DMEM w/o FBS. Combine PEI and DNA mix and incubate at room temperature for 15–30 min. Subsequently, add the transfection mix dropwise to the 293T/17 cells and place the culture dish into the incubator (*see* **Note 18**).
3. The next day, replace the medium with 7 ml DMEM with 10% FBS. After 24 h, collect the supernatant, with the help of a syringe pass it through a 0.45 μm PES filter into a 50 ml Falcon tube and store at 4 °C. Add 7 ml fresh DMEM with 10% FBS

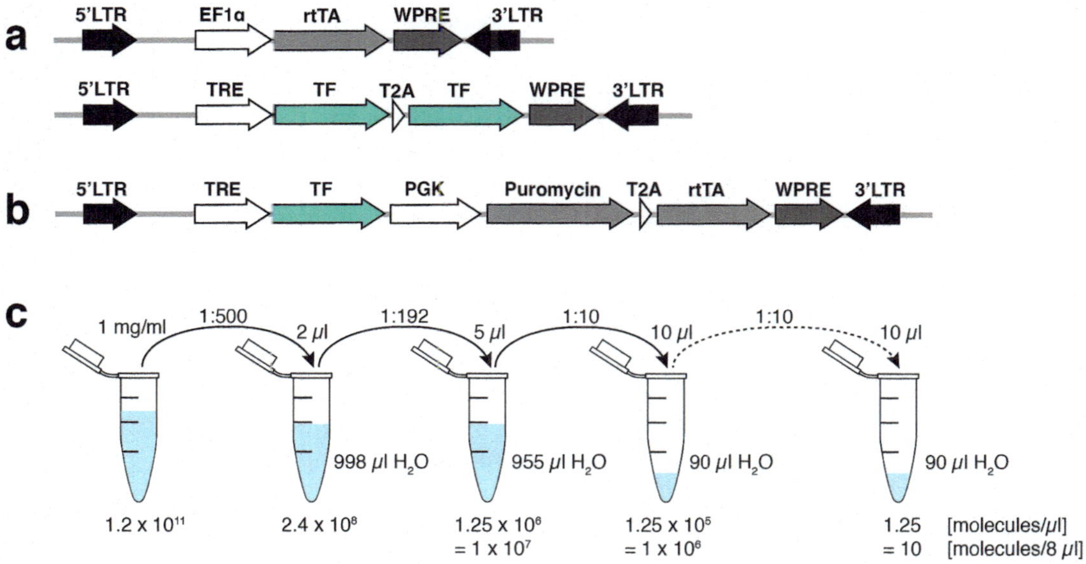

Fig. 3 Transduction of iPSCs with lentiviral vectors. (**a**) and (**b**) Schematic representation of the lentiviral constructs. (**a**) The pLV system consists of two constructs: pLV_hEF1a_rtTA3 (top) expresses the rtTA transactivator under the control of the constitutively active EF1α promoter and pLV_TRET_Ngn2-2A-Ngn1 (bottom) expresses the transgenes under the control of the doxycycline-inducible TRE promotor [4]. The pLV plasmids depicted to here do not contain any selection markers. If selection is required, antibiotic resistance genes should be cloned into the plasmids. (**b**) The pLIX403 system is an "all-in-one" doxycycline-inducible system. It expresses a puromycin resistance gene together with the rtTA transactivator under the control of the constitutively active PGK promotor and the transgene under the control of the doxycycline-inducible TRE promotor. 5′ and 3′ LTR—long terminal repeats, WPRE—woodchuck hepatitis virus posttranscriptional regulatory element. (**c**) Schematic representation of the serial dilution of the pAlbumin plasmid for titration and copy number determination (modified from [8])

and after another 24 h collect the supernatant, filter and pool with the first collection.

4. Mix 14 ml of cell culture supernatant (48 h and 72 h harvests) with 6.6 ml of diluted polyethyleneglycol (PEG) solution containing 3.5 ml of 50% PEG 6000 solution, 1.5 ml of 4 M NaCl solution, and 1.6 ml of 1× PBS w/o Ca^{2+} and Mg^{2+}, and keep at 4 °C overnight or over the weekend. Centrifuge the tubes at 7000 g for 10 min at 4 °C (*see* **Note 19**). After the centrifugation, a white pellet should be visible. Carefully decant the supernatant and resuspend the pellet in 150 µl 1× PBS w/o Ca^{2+} and Mg^{2+} by pipetting up and down. Vigorously vortex the tubes for 20–30 s to further resuspend the pellets. Lenti-X™ GoStix™ can be used to confirm the successful generation of viral particles. Transfer the virus suspension into 1.5 ml screw-cap tubes in aliquots of 50 µl, snap-freeze in crushed dry ice and store at −80 °C.
5. In order to transfect iPSCs with the viral particles, the cells should be approximately 40 ± 10% confluent. Wash the cells

once with 1× PBS w/o Ca^{2+} and Mg^{2+} and add mTeSR™1 medium to the well. Add mTeSR™1 to the tube containing the virus suspension, mix gently and transfer dropwise to one or more wells (*see* **Note 20**). Incubate the culture dish overnight and change the medium on the next day (*see* **Note 21**). Starting 48 h after transduction, select for cells with an integrated construct with the appropriate antibiotic (*see* **Note 14**).

6. For titration and copy number determination, we perform a qPCR on genomic DNA to count the number of integrated viral particles (WPRE) relative to the genome (albumin gene). Wait at least 96 h before isolating genomic DNA using a genomic DNA extraction kit, such as the DNeasy® Blood and Tissue Kit (Qiagen), according to the manufacturer's instructions. The DNA should be placed on ice if used immediately or stored at −20 °C.
7. Adjust the concentration of the pAlbumin plasmid used for normalization to 1 mg/ml, which corresponds to 1.2×10^{11} molecules/μl (*see* **Note 22**). Prepare a standard curve, with the first point being 1×10^7 molecules in 8 μl (which corresponds to 1.25×10^6 molecules/μl). Prepare the other points of the standard curve by serial tenfold dilutions until there are ten molecules in 8 μl (*see* Fig. 3c).
8. Prepare two master mixes of 8.5 μl TaqMan® Universal PCR Master Mix, 0.17 μl forward primer (10 μM), 0.17 μl reverse primer (10 μM), and 0.17 μl probe (10 μM) per sample including all samples and standards in duplicates (one master mix with albumin primers and probe for genomic DNA detection and one with WPRE primers and probe for lentivirus detection). Aliquot 9 μl master mix per well of a 96-well plate and add 8 μl of sample DNA (concentration between 50 and 100 ng DNA in 8 μl). Seal the plate, carefully mix by vortexing and briefly spin down. Run the qPCR with the settings for FAM fluorochromes and BHQ quenchers with the following program: 1 cycle of 10 min at 95 °C followed by 50 cycles of 15 s at 95 °C and 1 min at 60 °C (*see* **Note 17**).
9. Plot the standard curve using the software of your qPCR machine or manually using other software such as Microsoft Excel, and calculate the quantity of albumin and WPRE for each sample using the equation of the standard curve.
10. Calculate the copy number for each sample as follows: Copy number = (quantity mean of WPRE sequence/quantity mean of Alb sequence) × 2.
11. Calculate the viral titer with the following formula: Titer (viral genome/ml) = (number of target cells counted at day 1 × number of copies per cell of the sample)/volume of supernatant (ml).

3.4 Genome Editing with CRISPR/Cas9

1. Design a sgRNA for the locus of interest using designing tools (such as http://crispr.mit.edu/, *see* **Note 23**) [12].
2. Order two oligos representing the sgRNA with a design as follows: top oligo—CACC(G)[20 N of sgRNA], bottom oligo—AAAC[20 N reverse complement of sgRNA](C) [10] (*see* **Note 24**).
3. Anneal the oligos in a thermocycler using 2 μl top oligo, 2 μl bottom oligo, 2 μl 10× T4 Ligation Buffer, T4 Polynucleotide Kinase, and 13 μl ddH_2O and program the thermocycler with 30 min at 37 °C, 5 min at 95 °C, a ramp down to 25 °C (ramp rate of 5 °C/min) and hold at 4 °C. The oligo hybrid can directly be used for cloning into the linearized PX459 or PX458 vector.
4. Cut and dephosphorylate the vector using 2 μl BbsI with 3 μg of vector and fill up to 50 μl reaction volume with ddH_2O (minimum of 0.5 μl BbsI for 5 μg of vector). Incubate for 1 h at 37 °C and optionally heat-inactivate the digestion for 15 min at 65 °C. Gel-purify the vector by running on an agarose gel and extracting the band using a gel extraction kit, such as QIAquick® Gel Extraction Kit (Qiagen), according to the manufacturer's instructions. The vector can be stored at −20 °C for several months.
5. Ligate sgRNA insert and vector in a 10 μl reaction with 100 ng vector, 2 μl of the oligo hybrid (1:250 diluted), 5 μl Mighty Mix, and ddH_2O. Incubate the mixture for 30 min at 16 °C.
6. Transform 5 μl of the reaction product into chemically competent bacteria, such as Stbl3. The rest of the reaction can be stored for up to 2 weeks. Thaw the bacteria for ~10 min on ice, add the ligation reaction, stir carefully and incubate on ice for 5–10 min. Perform a heat shock for 45 s at 42 °C transfer the sample back to ice for 2–5 min. Add 300 μl S.O.C. medium and shake the bacteria for 1 h at 37 °C and 300 rpm. Plate the bacteria on LB-plates with 100 μg/ml ampicillin and incubate overnight at 37 °C and proceed with the plasmid preparation using a Miniprep kit such as the QIAprep® Spin Miniprep Kit (Qiagen) according to the manufacturer's guidelines.
7. Check the construct for correctness using the respective sequencing primer and expand the DNA to a high concentration stock. Optionally: Test the cutting efficiency with a T7 endonuclease assay [13] (*see* **Note 25**).
8. If homologous recombination of a disease correction or knockin of a reporter is the aim of the gene editing, a donor construct has to be provided in addition to the Cas9-sgRNA vector(s). The tag or the gene for the knockin should be framed by regions of the locus in approximately the same length as the part that is transferred into the gene (such as

~1000 bp for incorporation of an antibiotic resistance with promoter) and provided as a linearized DNA fragment. Alternatively, 5–25 bp homology can be used with microhomology-mediated end-joining [14].

9. Electroporate 10 μg of the vector encoding for the correct sgRNA and optionally ~5 μg of donor construct into iPSCs (*see* Subheadings 2.2 and 3.2). Seed the cells into two wells of a 6-well plate.
10. Using the PX459 vector, it is advisable to use 0.5–0.8 μg/ml puromycin for 12–16 h for the next night after electroporation in combination with ROCKi.
11. Keep ROCKi for 2 days and check if you obtained single cells that grow to small colonies. Once the colonies are visible by eye, check half of a colony for integration or knockout of the target gene by (colony) PCR with primers binding around or in the locus that you tested for specificity before (using control DNA). Transfer the other part of each colony not used for PCR to a new well (of a 48-well plate). These are the monoclonal knockout lines usable if the PCR shows the respective shifts.
12. Once a potentially positive clone has been detected, sequence the locus using Sanger sequencing, optimally with subcloning of the PCR product into a carrier vector (for instance using TOPO cloning).

3.5 Doxycycline-Induced Differentiation

1. Neurons can be grown on Matrigel-coated cell culture dishes, however, especially for long-term neuronal differentiation, it is recommended to grow the neurons on cell culture plates coated with poly-L-lysine (PLL) and laminin. Dilute the PLL in ddH_2O to a final concentration of 40 μg/ml, add the diluted PLL solution to the cell culture plates and distribute equally so that the entire well is covered. Incubate at 37 °C overnight and wash three times with ddH_2O on the next day. Dilute the laminin in 1× PBS with Ca^{2+} and Mg^{2+} to a final concentration of 20 μg/ml and add to the PLL-coated cell culture plates. Incubate at 37 °C for approximately 4 h. Prior to use, simply aspirate the coating solution and seed the cells without washing the plates.
2. Seed the iPSCs at a density of 30,000–50,000 cells per cm^2 in mTeSR™1 medium with ROCKi supplemented with 0.5 μg/ml doxycycline. On the next day, wash the cells with 1× PBS w/o Ca^{2+} and Mg^{2+} and change the medium to mTeSR™1 w/o ROCKi supplemented with 0.5 μg/ml doxycycline. Change the medium daily until day 4 (Fig. 4).
3. When culturing the neurons for longer time periods, it is recommended to change the stem cell medium (mTeSR™1) to maturation medium (BrainPhys™ with supplements).

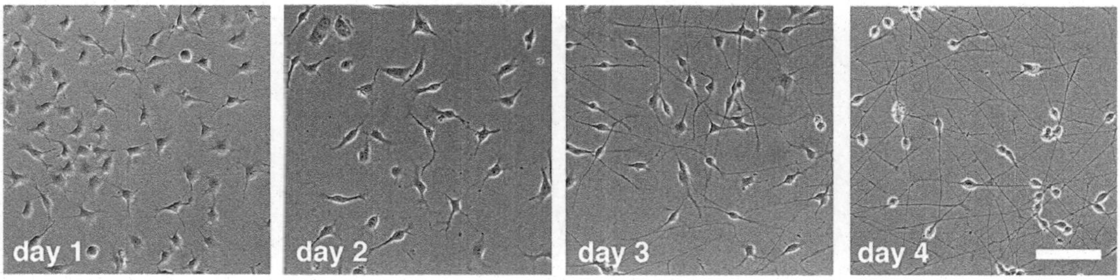

Fig. 4 Representative images of neuronal differentiation of human iPSCs expressing the neurogenic TFs Neurogenin-1 and Neurogenin-2 (iNGN cells) under the control of a doxycycline-inducible promoter [4]. Scale bar represents 100 μm

Change half of the medium on day 5 of differentiation to BrainPhys™ medium with supplements. Repeat changing half of the medium 2 days later. After those two adaptation medium changes, it is sufficient to change half of the medium once per week. Volume loss due to evaporation should be compensated with ddH_2O.

3.6 Coculturing with Astrocytes

1. In order to increase the maturation of neurons for electrophysiological measurements, coculturing with astrocytes is highly recommended [4, 15]. We adapted the protocol from Kaech and Banker [16] to our cell culture.
2. Rat primary cortical astrocytes are cultured in astrocyte medium at 37 °C and 5% CO_2 according to the manufacturer's instructions. For passaging, aspirate the culture medium and store it in a Falcon tube as a washing solution (*see* **Note 26**). Rinse the cells once with 1× PBS w/o Ca^{2+} and Mg^{2+}. Add prewarmed Accutase and incubate the cells at 37 °C until all of them are detached (usually 5 min are sufficient). Stepwise add the cell culture medium stored in the first step to flush cells and collect all cells to a prerinsed 15 ml Falcon tube. Centrifuge at 400 × *g* for 5 min. Aspirate the supernatant and resuspend the pellet in prewarmed astrocyte growth medium. Count the cells using Trypan Blue and seed the appropriate amount in uncoated tissue-culture treated dishes at a seeding density of approximately 5000 cells per cm^2. Change the growth medium every 3–4 days.
3. For the coculture with neurons, prepare astrocytes to be ~80% confluent at day 4 of neuronal differentiation. One day before the reseeding of neurons, wash the astrocytes three times with 1× PBS w/o Ca^{2+} and Mg^{2+} and add BrainPhys™ medium with minimal supplements.
4. Thoroughly clean the coverslips in a big glass petri dish. First, rinse the coverslips in ddH_2O for 2 h and then shake in 50 ml

1 M HCl overnight. Rinse three times with ddH_2O by shaking for 2 min, and rinse another two times with ddH_2O by shaking for 2 h. Shake three times in 100% ethanol for 2 min and one time overnight. Sterilize the coverslips at 225 °C for 6–16 h (can be done overnight) (*see* **Note 27**) [16].

5. Autoclave ~100 ml low melting paraffin in a 500 ml bottle. Melt in a boiling water bath (1 l beaker with 400 ml H_2O on a heat plate with 350 °C). Use a 2 ml aspiration pipette with a 200 μl pipette tip attached and soak it in melted paraffin. Shake off extra drops and place small drops on coverslips to create paraffin feet as spacer (*see* **Note 28**). Coat the coverslips with PLL and laminin (*see* Subheading 3.5) on the side with the paraffin dots.
6. Differentiate the iPSCs on Matrigel-coated cell culture dishes using 0.5 μg/ml doxycycline in mTeSR™1 medium for 4 days (*see* Subheading 3.5). Add 5 μM Ara-C to the culture for 1 day to remove occasionally undifferentiated cells.
7. At day 5, reseed predifferentiated neurons on PLL and laminin coated coverslips with paraffin feet. Collect the old medium from the culture well and wash the cells very carefully with prewarmed 1× PBS w/o Ca^{2+}, Mg^{2+}. Dissociate the cells by adding Accutase and place in the incubator for approximately 5 min until the neuronal network detaches. Add the cell culture medium stored in the first step and transfer the cell solution to a 15 ml Falcon tube. Rinse the well 1–2 times with 1% BSA to collect all cells and centrifuge at 400 × *g* for 5 min. Aspirate the supernatant and resuspend the cell pellet in 200 μl 0.2% BSA slowly and carefully (this step is crucial for the survival of single cells). Add 800 μl of 0.2% BSA to a total volume of 1 ml. Centrifuge at 20 × *g* for 1 min and collect 800 μl supernatant in a fresh tube (this is the single cell suspension). Repeat the dissociation of the pellet for a maximum of five times until no pellet is visible any more. Centrifuge the single cell suspension at 400 × *g* for 5 min and resuspend the pellet in 0.5 ml BrainPhys™ medium. Count the cells if necessary and seed on coated coverslips on the side with the paraffin feet (*see* **Note 29**).
8. After 2 h, place the coverslips with the differentiated iPSCs upside down into culture wells containing 80% confluent rat astrocytes. Every 7 days, exchange 50% of the BrainPhys™ medium and compensate the volume loss due to evaporation with ddH_2O (*see* **Note 30**).

4 Notes

1. Aliquot the Matrigel according to the protocol and the dilution factor provided with it (varies for each bottle of Matrigel). We prepare aliquots for dilution in 12 ml coating medium. Briefly, thaw the Matrigel on ice in the cold room or the fridge and prepare a box with dry ice to precool 1.5 ml tubes. Quickly distribute the Matrigel solution into the tubes and store at −20 °C.
2. The piggyBac vector backbone can be obtained from Addgene (to be submitted, containing the EGFP gene under the control of the doxycycline-inducible promoter). For cloning of transcription factors, the EGFP can be excised using NheI and XhoI, the transcription factor cDNA can be amplified by PCR and introduced into the piggyBac vector using Gibson Assembly cloning [17].
3. There are two different lentiviral vector systems that can be used: the pLV system that consists of two constructs, one expressing the rtTA transactivator from the constitutively active EF1α promoter and the other one expressing the transgene under the control of the doxycycline-inducible TRE promoter [4] (Addgene plasmids #61472 and #61471, respectively) or the pLIX403 system that expresses the rtTA transactivator and the transgene under the TRE promoter on a single construct (Addgene plasmid #41395). The pLV plasmids that are referred to in this protocol do not contain any selection markers. If selection for the integrated constructs is required, it should be cloned into the plasmids before the production of lentiviral particles.
4. For better attachment of the neurons, freshly add 1 μl of a 1 mg/ml laminin solution per 1 ml supplemented BrainPhys™ medium to a final concentration of 1 μg/ml.
5. For the coculture with astrocytes, we use BrainPhys™ medium with a minimal supplementation since we found that astrocytes do not grow well in the presence of cAMP. Addition of BDNF and GDNF was neither found to enhance maturation nor affect astrocytes but might be beneficial depending on experiment design.
6. Use 1 ml of diluted Matrigel solution per well of a 6-well plate, 0.5 ml per well of a 12-well plate and 0.25 ml per well of a 24-well plate.
7. Use 2 ml mTeSR™1 medium per well of a 6-well plate, 1 ml per well of a 12-well plate and 0.5 ml per well of a 24-well plate. If you would like to avoid feeding the cells on the weekend, add at least the 1.5-fold amount of medium on Friday.

8. The optimal cell density depends on the growth rate of your iPSC line. For our cells, we seed 15,000–25,000 cells/cm^2 for maintenance of stem cells, and 30,000–50,000 cells/cm^2 for differentiation experiments.
9. Check iPSCs in 4-week intervals for mycoplasma contamination using the Universal Mycoplasma Detection Kit (ATCC® 30-1012K™) according to the manufacturer's instructions.
10. The optimal density for freezing depends on your iPSC line. For our cells, a density of 500,000–1,000,000 cells/cryotube in 0.5–1 ml mFreSR™ works well.
11. Cells of one 100 μl nucleofection reaction can be seeded to one well of a 6-well plate or distributed to multiple wells of a 12- or 24-well plate.
12. The pulse CB-156 is recommended if higher transfection efficiency is favored at expenses of a lower survival rate, whereas the pulse CB-150 results in higher viability with lower transfection efficiency.
13. Leaving the cells in Nucleofector™ solution for extended periods of time may lead to reduced transfection efficiency and viability so it is important to work as quickly as possible. If you face problems such as low transfection efficiency due to very big plasmids etc. you can try to incubate the cells after nucleofection in the Nucleofector™ solution at room temperature for approximately 10 min.
14. The concentration of antibiotic optimal for selection depends on the specific iPSC line of choice and should be determined with a killing curve. We use a final concentration of 20 μg/ml for blasticidin, 3 μg/ml for puromycin, and 250 μg/ml for hygromycin.
15. Alternatively, the copy number can be determined as described for the lentiviral transduction (*see* Subheading 3.3) by performing a TaqMan®-based qPCR on genomic DNA. Use the albumin gene for normalization and a gene specific for the piggyBac construct for counting the integration events. We recommend using primers and probes for the antibiotic resistance gene, if not otherwise present in the genome of your iPSC line. It is important to have both genes present on the same plasmid used for the standard curve since the preparation of the serial dilutions is prone to small variations.
16. Before performing the copy number determination, the cells must be passaged at least once to avoid the interference of nonintegrated piggyBac plasmids with the qPCR.
17. The optimal settings of the qPCR protocol may vary with the qPCR machine and the SYBR® Green or TaqMan® mix used. The settings described in this protocol are referring to the StepOnePlus™Real-Time PCR System (Thermo Fisher

Scientific), with the Power SYBR® Green PCR Master Mix (Thermo Fisher Scientific) or the TaqMan® Universal PCR Master Mix (Thermo Fisher Scientific).

18. From this step on, the cells are producing viral particles and should be handled at biosafety level 2. All viral particles that are collected are also biosafety level 2.
19. If your centrifuge is not able to run at 7000 × *g*, the centrifugation step can be carried out at lower g for a longer period of time (e.g., at 5000 × *g* for 30 min).
20. We usually use one aliquot of viral particles to transduce one well of a 6- or 12-well plate. In order to optimize the viral transduction, it is recommended to determine the viral titer. Therefore, transduce cells with different volumes of the virus-containing supernatant and perform a qPCR on genomic DNA counting the number of integrated copies per cell.
21. Directly after transfection, the iPSCs are biosafety level 2 and should be handled as such, after the medium change the next day, they are back at biosafety level 1.
22. The calculation of the molecule number per μl in a solution with a concentration of 1 mg/ml is as follows: molecules/μl = (6.022 × 10^{23} 1/mol [Avogadro constant]/(length of the plasmid × 660 Da [average molecular weight of a base pair])) × 10^{-6} g/μl. For the pAlbumin plasmid with a length of 7539 bp, the calculation is: (6.022 × 10^{23} 1/mol/(7539 bp × 660 Da)) × 10^{-6} g/μl = 1.2 × 10^{11} molecules/μl.
23. Avoid placing the PAM sequence into your sgRNA-expressing vector and the potential donor construct. It will be cut once sgRNA and Cas9 are expressed. The vectors from the Zhang lab can be ordered in different versions, that is, with GFP or puromycin expression. If positive cells should be sorted with flow cytometry, GFP is optimal. When expanding of single cells and subsequent picking of monoclonal colonies is preferred, use puromycin with the version V2 on Addgene, which is corrected from a previous version. The success rate of this cloning strategy is usually very high.
24. One or two guanines can be added for more efficiency of the U6 promoter if the designed sgRNA is not starting with it. They have to be added to the bottom oligo as reverse complement in addition to the sgRNA sequence as well.
25. The T7 endonuclease I assay is performed as follows: Transfect the sgRNA- and Cas9-expressing constructs into a test cell line (e.g., 293T/17, *see* Subheadings 2.3 and 3.3). Isolate the DNA using a DNA extraction kit, such as the DNeasy® Blood and Tissue Kit (Qiagen). Amplify the locus using flanking primers tested for specificity in advance. Purify the reaction

using a PCR Purification kit (Qiagen). Elute in 30 µl. Mix 200 ng purified PCR product, 2 µl NEBuffer™ 2 and water to a total volume of 19 µl. Hybridize the PCR product in a thermocycler by heating to 95 °C and ramp down to 85 °C with −2 °C/s, then to 25 °C with 0.1 °C/s and hold at 4 °C. Add 1 µl T7 endonuclease I to the reaction and incubate at 37 °C for 20 min. Run on a 2% agarose gel (30 min, 90 V) to see if one or more bands appear. If two or three bands are visible, the sgRNA works fine. The T7 endonuclease cuts at wobbles that appear with reannealing of nonfitting DNA [13] strands. This happens if the Cas9 cuts parts of the DNA of the population of cells used as the test cell line.

26. Rat Primary Cortical Astrocytes stick to the plastic used in cell culture dishes and centrifuge tubes. Prior to use, rinse all material that will come in contact with the cells with medium to prevent cells from sticking to the plastic.
27. Since the cleaning of the coverslips is very time-consuming, it can also be done in 1 day. Briefly, rinse the coverslips two times in ddH_2O, then add 50 ml 1 M HCl and shake for 1 h. Rinse three times with ddH_2O by shaking for 2 min, and then rinse once more with ddH_2O by shaking for 1 h. Shake three times in 100% ethanol for 2 min and one time for 1 h. Sterilize the coverslips at 225 °C for 2–3 h. Successful cleaning will be accompanied by an even spread of coating solution across the whole surface of the coverslip. If problems with adhesion occur, go back to the long protocol.
28. The purpose of the spacers is to allow growth of the induced neurons in close proximity to the astrocyte feeder layer but without physical contact.
29. The coverslips can have any size depending on the requirements of the experiment. We routinely use 12 mm coverslips equipped with three paraffin feet in a 24-well plate. It is recommended to add additional volume of medium to the well to completely cover the coverslips in order to avoid floating.
30. We add approximately 50 µl ddH_2O per week for a 24-well plate to compensate for volume loss due to evaporation. Store a test plate full of H_2O in the incubator and weigh in weekly intervals to check for evaporation.

Acknowledgments

This work was supported by Volkswagen Foundation Freigeist fellowship A110720 and ERC starting grant 678071—ProNeurons to V.B. E.J.S. and L.K.K. were supported by the DIGS-BB PhD Program.

References

1. Srikanth P, Young-Pearse TL (2014) Stem cells on the brain: modeling neurodevelopmental and neurodegenerative diseases using human induced pluripotent stem cells. J Neurogenet 28:5–29
2. Shi Y, Inoue H, Wu JC, Yamanaka S (2017) Induced pluripotent stem cell technology: a decade of progress. Nat Rev Drug Discov 16:115–130
3. Doudna JA, Charpentier E (2014) Genome editing. The new frontier of genome engineering with CRISPR-Cas9. Science 346:1258096
4. Busskamp V et al (2014) Rapid neurogenesis through transcriptional activation in human stem cells. Mol Syst Biol 10:760
5. Chanda S et al (2014) Generation of induced neuronal cells by the single reprogramming factor ASCL1. Stem Cell Reports 3:282–296
6. Yang N et al (2017) Generation of pure GABAergic neurons by transcription factor programming. Nat Methods 14:621–628
7. Zhang Y et al (2013) Rapid single-step induction of functional neurons from human pluripotent stem cells. Neuron 78:785–798
8. Barde I, Salmon P, Trono D (2010) Production and titration of lentiviral vectors. Curr Protoc Neurosci. Chapter 4, Unit 4 21
9. Zhao S et al (2016) PiggyBac transposon vectors: the tools of the human gene encoding. Transl Lung Cancer Res 5:120–125
10. Ran FA et al (2013) Genome engineering using the CRISPR-Cas9 system. Nat Protoc 8:2281–2308
11. Livak KJ, Schmittgen TD (2001) Analysis of relative gene expression data using real-time quantitative PCR and the 2(−Delta Delta C (T)) method. Methods 25:402–408
12. Hsu PD et al (2013) DNA targeting specificity of RNA-guided Cas9 nucleases. Nat Biotechnol 31:827–832
13. Guschin DY et al (2010) A rapid and general assay for monitoring endogenous gene modification. Methods Mol Biol 649:247–256
14. Sakuma T, Nakade S, Sakane Y, Suzuki KT, Yamamoto T (2016) MMEJ-assisted gene knock-in using TALENs and CRISPR-Cas9 with the PITCh systems. Nat Protoc 11:118–133
15. Lam RS, Topfer FM, Wood PG, Busskamp V, Bamberg E (2017) Functional maturation of human stem cell-derived neurons in long-term cultures. PLoS One 12:e0169506
16. Kaech S, Banker G (2006) Culturing hippocampal neurons. Nat Protoc 1:2406–2415
17. Gibson DG (2011) Enzymatic assembly of overlapping DNA fragments. Methods Enzymol 498:349–361

Chapter 10

Imaging of Somatic Ca^{2+} Transients in Differentiated Human Neurons

Irena Vertkin and Dalit Ben-Yosef

Abstract

Calcium is a major regulator of neuronal activity and calcium signaling is critically important for normal neuronal function. Ca imaging is a well-established tool for studying neuronal function and ongoing spontaneous Ca^{2+} transients are a good indicator of neuronal maturity. There are various indicators available today, differing by their sensitivity, spectra, and loading method. Here we present a method for measurement of Ca^{2+} transients in neurons using two different Ca^{2+} indicators, Oregon Green BAPTA-1 and GCaMP6.

Key words Human induced pluripotent stem cells, Somatic Ca^{2+} transients, Calcium indicators, Oregon Green-488 BAPTA-1AM, GCaMP6

1 Introduction

Calcium ions are one of the main mediators of cellular activity that regulate large variety of functions in all types of cells ranging from gene expression to cell proliferation and cell death [1–3]. In neuronal cells calcium signaling regulates neuronal activity, such as release of neurotransmitters, synaptic plasticity and excitability in spatiotemporal manner [4–7]. That is why intracellular calcium signaling is one of the major targets in studying neuronal function [8–10].

At the rest state, neurons maintain low levels of intracellular Ca^{2+}. During neuronal activity increasing depolarization of the membrane triggers opening of the voltage dependent Ca^{2+} channels, causing significant increase in intracellular Ca^{2+} which in turn causes variety of processes, such as neurotransmitter release [1, 11]. Eventually, the excess of intracellular Ca^{2+} is cleared by the buffering action of cytosolic Ca^{2+}-binding proteins and by its uptake by mitochondria [3, 12, 13]. The inability of neurons to maintain normal Ca^{2+} signaling is one of the hallmarks of various neurological diseases [14–17].

Dalit Ben-Yosef and Yoav Mayshar (eds.), *Fragile-X Syndrome: Methods and Protocols*, Methods in Molecular Biology, vol. 1942, https://doi.org/10.1007/978-1-4939-9080-1_10, © Springer Science+Business Media, LLC, part of Springer Nature 2019

First Ca^{2+} indicators were developed by Tsien over 30 years ago [18]. Currently a large variety of Ca^{2+} indicators exist differing in their properties, such as affinity for Ca^{2+} or excitation–emission spectra [19, 20]. There are two major families of Ca^{2+} indicators used today in research. First is the family of chemical calcium indicators, which are based on calcium chelator molecule conjugated to the fluorophore [20]. In the absence of Ca^{2+}, photo-induced electron transfer from the Ca^{2+} chelator quenches fluorescence of the conjugated fluorophore. As Ca^{2+} levels rise the binding of Ca^{2+} ions causes conformational changes, leading to an increase in fluorescence intensity. Here we describe use of Oregon Green BAPTA-1 (OGB1), one of the indicators belonging to this family of chemical indicators. It has very high sensitivity, can detect fast Ca^{2+} signals and has very good signal to noise ratio. Recently, a second family of calcium indicators has been developed, genetically encoded fluorescent Ca^{2+} indicators (GECIs). One kind of GECI is based on two fluorophores where Ca^{2+} binding effects Förster resonance energy transfer (FRET) between them. Another kind of GECI is a GCaMP family of single-fluorophore sensors consisting of the circularly permuted green fluorescent protein (GFP) linked to the calmodulin (CaM) binding region of myosin light kinase (M13) at its N terminus, and to a CaM at its C terminus [21, 22]. In the presence of calcium the M13 and CaM domains interact causing conformational change which results in increased fluorescence. Here we also describe use of recently developed GCaMP6 indicator, which has good sensitivity and wide dynamic range [23].

Recently, calcium imaging is becoming a successful alternative tool for electrophysiology to monitor neuronal activity in large population of neurons. It can be used to evaluate mean firing rate and patterns of spiking activity since there is a correlation between them. Here, we use calcium imaging to study neuronal activity in differentiated human neurons.

2 Materials

2.1 Preparation of Neuronal Culture for Imaging

1. Differentiated neurons grown in 24-well plate or on coverslips (*see* **Note 1**).
2. 1 mM Oregon Green-488 BAPTA-1AM (OGB) (Invitrogen) stock: dissolve 50 μg (entire vial) in 39.74 μl of DMSO.
3. GCaMP6 plasmid DNA.
4. Lipofectamine 2000 (Invitrogen).
5. BrainPhys Neuronal medium (STEMCELLS)—preincubate at 37°C and 5% CO_2 (*see* **Note 2**).
6. Tyrode solution: 145 mM NaCl; 3 mM KCl; 15 mM glucose; 10 mM Hepes; 1.2 mM MgCl2; 1.2 mM $CaCl_2$, pH adjusted

to 7.4 with NaOH. Tyrode solution can be used at room temperature.

2.2 Imaging Acquisition

1. Imaging microscope.
2. Microscope stagetop incubator with CO_2 supply and temperature controller (*see* **Note 3**).

2.3 Data Analysis

1. Image processing software (such as ImageJ).
2. Statistical software (such as GraphPad Prism).

3 Methods

3.1 Preparation of Neuronal Culture for Imaging

3.1.1 Calcium Green-488 BAPTA-1AM (OGB) Loading

1. Remove medium from the well and add 0.5 ml of fresh preincubated BrainPhys medium, add 1.5 μl of 1 mM OGB solution to the final concentration of 3 μM.
2. Incubate for 30 min at 37°C and 5% CO_2.
3. Remove OGB solution and add 0.5–1 ml of fresh preincubated BrainPhys or Tyrode solution and transfer cells to the imaging microscope (*see* **Note 4**).

3.1.2 GCaMP6 Transfection

1. Prepare two tubes with BrainPhys medium, suggested volume is 50–75 μl per well of 24-well plate in each tube. To the first tube add required amount of DNA, usually 1–2 μg per well, to the second tube add Lipofectamine 2000, suggested volume is 2 μl per 1 μg of DNA. Incubate for 5 min at room temperature. Mix the two tubes. We usually transfer Lipofectamine solution into DNA mix while gently vortexing the DNA tube. Incubate for 20 min at room temperature.
2. Remove medium from the cells, add 350–400 μl of preincubated BrainPhys medium to each well. Then add transfection mix, 100–150 μl per well to the final volume of 500 μl per well. Incubate for 30 min at 37°C and 5% CO_2.
3. Remove transfection mix from the cells, wash cells carefully with 1 ml of preincubated BrainPhys medium, and add 0.5–1 ml of fresh preincubated BrainPhys medium.
4. Cells can be imaged after 24–48 h following transfection (*see* **Note 5**).

3.2 Image Acquisition

1. Mount plate with cells under the microscope. For imaging in usual cell medium, a stagetop incubator with heating and CO_2 supply is required. Imaging in Tyrode solution can be done at room temperature (*see* **Notes 6** and 7).
2. Select region of interest. Adjust image acquisition parameters (intensity of excitation lamp and exposure time should be

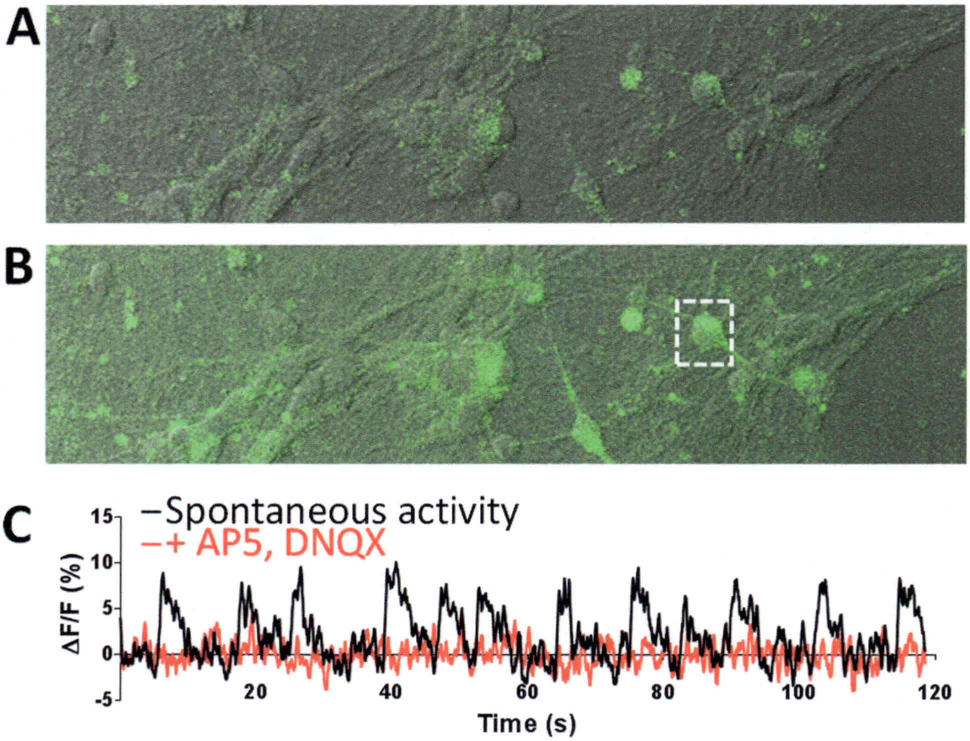

Fig. 1 Somatic Ca^{2+} transients in iN. iN (48 days post-induction) loaded with OGB-488 during rest period (**A**) and during spike activity (**B**). (**C**) Recording of changes in somatic Ca^{2+} level in single neuron during spontaneous activity, activity severely decreases after addition of glutamate receptors blockers (AP5, DNQX)

adjusted to get clear signal without causing bleaching and phototoxicity) (*see* **Note 8**). Adjust experimental parameters (frequency of the imaging acquisition needs to be as high as possible, but at least around 10–20 Hz) (*see* **Note 9**). Take images for 2 min, and wait for 10–15 min to let the cells rest. Repeat imaging the required number of times. If possible, other regions or wells can be imaged during rest time (*see* **Note 10**). Figure 1 demonstrates bright field image of human induced neurons (iN) loaded with OGB-488 during rest period (A) and during neuronal activity (B). There is a visible increase in fluorescence caused by an increase in intracellular Ca^{2+}.

3. For GFP based Ca^{2+}indicator, imaging is performed by using excitation wavelength of 488 nm. Emission is detected between 510 and 570 nm.

3.3 Image Analysis

1. Open image sequence in image processing software, select regions of interest (ROI) by drawing outline of cell soma.
2. Calculate fluorescence intensity values for each time point. Transfer data to analysis software program.

3. Normalize data to baseline. Calculate frequency, maximal amplitude and area under the curve for each peak. Figure 1C demonstrates typical recording of Ca^{2+} transients in the selected neuron, normalized to baseline (fluorescence intensity during rest period).

4 Notes

1. Depending on the experiment, neurons can be grown directly in 24-well plate wells or on coverslip. If observation of cultures is required for a prolonged period of time, direct growth on the plate is preferential. For short experiments coverslips may be used, because only one coverslip is moved to microscope without disturbing the entire plate. Importantly, the plastic plates commonly used for tissue culture, can decrease quality of the imaging due to their thickness and optic properties, and often require special lenses to accommodate for focus working distance. There are special imaging plates commercially available with glass bottoms for superior imaging.
2. Differentiated neurons are very sensitive to environmental factors. To preserve their function it is critical to decrease possible perturbations during the experiment. Most of the cellular mediums contain sodium bicarbonate which requires CO_2 to maintain physiological pH. Therefore, it is very important to preincubate experimental medium to equilibrate both temperature and pH. Since Tyrode solution is based on HEPES, it does not require prewarming. However, Tyrode solution is not recommended for human neurons.
3. While Ca^{2+} imaging can be performed at room temperature in Tyrode solution, neurons exhibit much more robust activity when imaging in growth medium. There are several commercially available models for stagetop incubators.
4. Concentration and time of OGB-488 incubation can be changed if required. Avoid prolong incubation because it can decrease signal-to-noise ratio. It is recommended to mix OGB-488 with medium by pipetting, since it is dissolved in DMSO and diffuses slowly if not mixed.
5. GECIs can be also delivered by viral vectors for high efficiency stable integration.
6. If there is weak or no fluorescence visible:
   (a) Instrument malfunction—check acquisition parameters, then perform imaging of the known fluorescent sample (can be purchased) to determine that microscope is functional.

(b) OGB-488—on very rare occurrences there is a poor loading, in that case it is recommended to use new cell sample or to prepare a new batch of OGB-488.

(c) GCaMP6—check for DNA degradation, try using higher DNA amounts. As well, control transfection with any fluorophore alone can be done simultaneously to ensure that there is no problem in transfection protocol.

7. Cells loaded or transfected with calcium indicator have basal fluorescence signal. While searching for appropriate regions of interest adjust acquisition parameters to be able to see weak fluorescence in the soma. If the signal in some neurons is very strong compared to the majority of the other cells it could indicate either neuronal death or overloading with indicator. Since indicator is a chelating agent, overloading usually results in blocking of Ca^{2+} signal. Thus, these overly bright cells should be avoided.
8. As mentioned in Methods, acquisition parameters should be selected to get the best image possible without excessive bleaching of fluorophore and damaging the cells. Usually we test several possible combinations of parameters and choose the one most appropriate for each specific experiment.
9. Action potentials induce sharp rises in florescence that usually take tens of milliseconds followed by slower decay. The peak amplitude is one of the parameters that give us the information about neuronal activity, so it is important to capture the peak of the increase. That is why the frequency of image acquisition needs to be sufficiently high not to miss the peak. The higher image acquisition rate usually better correlates with real spiking during neuronal activity, but it is limited by area of the region of interest and resolution. Acquisition rate 10–20 Hz rate can give us sufficiently good approximation of spiking neuronal activity.
10. Certain microscope setups offer possibility of storing the coordinates of ROI. Therefore, it is possible to record activity in other areas during rest periods in previously imaged ROI. It is important that ROI are sufficiently distant from each other, to avoid phototoxicity.

References

1. Berridge MJ, Lipp P, Bootman MD (2000) The versatility and universality of calcium signalling. Nat Rev Mol Cell Biol 1(1):11–21. https://doi.org/10.1038/35036035
2. Brini M, Cali T, Ottolini D, Carafoli E (2013) Intracellular calcium homeostasis and signaling. Met Ions Life Sci 12:119–168. https://doi.org/10.1007/978-94-007-5561-1_5
3. Berridge MJ, Bootman MD, Roderick HL (2003) Calcium signalling: dynamics, homeostasis and remodelling. Nat Rev Mol Cell Biol 4

(7):517–529. https://doi.org/10.1038/nrm1155

4. Tsien RW, Tsien RY (1990) Calcium channels, stores, and oscillations. Annu Rev Cell Biol 6:715–760. https://doi.org/10.1146/annurev.cb.06.110190.003435
5. Neher E (1998) Vesicle pools and Ca2– microdomains: new tools for understanding their roles in neurotransmitter release. Neuron 20 (3):389–399
6. Sudhof TC (2000) The synaptic vesicle cycle revisited. Neuron 28(2):317–320
7. Rusakov DA, Stewart MG, Korogod SM (1996) Branching of active dendritic spines as a mechanism for controlling synaptic efficacy. Neuroscience 75(1):315–323
8. Grienberger C, Konnerth A (2012) Imaging calcium in neurons. Neuron 73(5):862–885. https://doi.org/10.1016/j.neuron.2012.02.011
9. Kobayashi C, Ohkura M, Nakai J, Matsuki N, Ikegaya Y, Sasaki T (2014) Large-scale imaging of subcellular calcium dynamics of cortical neurons with G-CaMP6-actin. Neuroreport 25 (7):501–506. https://doi.org/10.1097/WNR.0000000000000126
10. Birkner A, Tischbirek CH, Konnerth A (2017) Improved deep two-photon calcium imaging in vivo. Cell Calcium 64:29–35. https://doi.org/10.1016/j.ceca.2016.12.005
11. Sudhof TC (2013) Neurotransmitter release: the last millisecond in the life of a synaptic vesicle. Neuron 80(3):675–690. https://doi.org/10.1016/j.neuron.2013.10.022
12. Duchen MR (1999) Contributions of mitochondria to animal physiology: from homeostatic sensor to calcium signalling and cell death. J Physiol 516. (Pt 1:1–17
13. Gazit N, Vertkin I, Shapira I, Helm M, Slomowitz E, Sheiba M, Mor Y, Rizzoli S, Slutsky I (2016) IGF-1 receptor differentially regulates spontaneous and evoked transmission via mitochondria at hippocampal synapses. Neuron 89(3):583–597. https://doi.org/10.1016/j.neuron.2015.12.034
14. Popugaeva E, Pchitskaya E, Bezprozvanny I (2017) Dysregulation of neuronal calcium homeostasis in Alzheimer's disease - a therapeutic opportunity? Biochem Biophys Res Commun 483(4):998–1004. https://doi.org/10.1016/j.bbrc.2016.09.053
15. Gleichmann M, Mattson MP (2011) Neuronal calcium homeostasis and dysregulation. Antioxid Redox Signal 14(7):1261–1273. https://doi.org/10.1089/ars.2010.3386
16. Zanni G, Cali T, Kalscheuer VM, Ottolini D, Barresi S, Lebrun N, Montecchi-Palazzi L, Hu H, Chelly J, Bertini E, Brini M, Carafoli E (2012) Mutation of plasma membrane Ca2+ ATPase isoform 3 in a family with X-linked congenital cerebellar ataxia impairs Ca2+ homeostasis. Proc Natl Acad Sci USA 109 (36):14514–14519. https://doi.org/10.1073/pnas.1207488109
17. Lim D, Fedrizzi L, Tartari M, Zuccato C, Cattaneo E, Brini M, Carafoli E (2008) Calcium homeostasis and mitochondrial dysfunction in striatal neurons of Huntington disease. J Biol Chem 283(9):5780–5789. https://doi.org/10.1074/jbc.M704704200
18. Tsien RY (1980) New calcium indicators and buffers with high selectivity against magnesium and protons: design, synthesis, and properties of prototype structures. Biochemistry 19 (11):2396–2404
19. Lock JT, Parker I, Smith IF (2015) A comparison of fluorescent Ca(2)(+) indicators for imaging local Ca(2)(+) signals in cultured cells. Cell Calcium 58(6):638–648. https://doi.org/10.1016/j.ceca.2015.10.003
20. Paredes RM, Etzler JC, Watts LT, Zheng W, Lechleiter JD (2008) Chemical calcium indicators. Methods 46(3):143–151. https://doi.org/10.1016/j.ymeth.2008.09.025
21. Hires SA, Tian L, Looger LL (2008) Reporting neural activity with genetically encoded calcium indicators. Brain Cell Biol 36 (1–4):69–86. https://doi.org/10.1007/s11068-008-9029-4
22. Tian L, Akerboom J, Schreiter ER, Looger LL (2012) Neural activity imaging with genetically encoded calcium indicators. Prog Brain Res 196:79–94. https://doi.org/10.1016/B978-0-444-59426-6.00005-7
23. Chen TW, Wardill TJ, Sun Y, Pulver SR, Renninger SL, Baohan A, Schreiter ER, Kerr RA, Orger MB, Jayaraman V, Looger LL, Svoboda K, Kim DS (2013) Ultrasensitive fluorescent proteins for imaging neuronal activity. Nature 499(7458):295–300. https://doi.org/10.1038/nature12354

Chapter 11

Patch-Clamp Recordings from Human Embryonic Stem Cells-Derived Fragile X Neurons

Michael Telias and Menahem Segal

Abstract

Performing electrophysiological recordings from human neurons that have been differentiated in vitro, as compared to primary cultures, raises many challenges. However, patch-clamp recording from neurons derived from stem cells provides an abundance of valuable information, reliably and fast. Here, we describe a protocol that is used successfully in our lab for recording from both control and Fragile X neurons, derived in vitro from human embryonic stem cells.

Key words Patch-clamp, Voltage-clamp, Current-clamp, Whole-cell, In vitro electrophysiological recording

1 Introduction

Neurodevelopmental disorders are the result of inherited or acquired impairments during the process of neurogenesis and/or synaptogenesis [1, 2]. Human embryonic or induced pluripotent stem cells (hESCs, hiPSCs), carrying specific mutations or derived from diagnosed patients, offer a unique opportunity to model human neurodevelopmental disorders in vitro [3, 4]. In such a line of research, an essential step is to study and characterize the electrophysiological properties of the differentiated neurons. Assessing these properties can shed light on the molecular and cellular mechanisms underlying the pathology in question, and provide insights into normal physiological processes responsible for neuronal and synaptic development [5, 6]. The "electrophysiological signature" of an in-vitro disease model can be used as a bioassay to evaluate the therapeutic potential of candidate drugs.

Many different methods exist to record the electrical activity of cells but here we will discuss the use of whole-cell patch-clamp [7]. In this method, a micropipette is used to directly record and control the cell membrane potential, which in turn produces an abundance of data on the passive and active properties of ionic

Dalit Ben-Yosef and Yoav Mayshar (eds.), *Fragile-X Syndrome: Methods and Protocols*, Methods in Molecular Biology, vol. 1942,
https://doi.org/10.1007/978-1-4939-9080-1_11,

currents, action potentials, synaptic currents, and more [8]. Patch-clamp recordings coupled with pharmacology can be used to characterize neuronal identity during and after differentiation; study the composition of receptors and their response, the properties of neurotransmitter secretion and the nature of synaptic transmission. However, carrying out whole-cell patch-clamp recordings on in vitro differentiated neurons is not trivial. Here, we summarize the main challenges to overcome, and offer some notes on how to do it.

2 Materials

2.1 Extracellular Recording Solution

Double-distilled water (DDW) containing 10 mM HEPES, 4 mM KCl, 2 mM $CaCl_2$, 1 mM $MgCl_2$, 139 mM NaCl, and 10 mM D-glucose. Adjust the pH of the solution to 7.4. Adjust the osmolality of the solution to 330 mOsm. The solution is kept in the refrigerator without $CaCl_2$ and $MgCl_2$, which are added before use. It is highly recommended to filter the solution, but since the procedure is not sterile, autoclaving the solution is not necessary. Warm up the solution to room temperature before use.

2.2 Intracellular Recording Solution

DDW containing: 136 mM K-gluconate, 10 mM KCl, 5 mM NaCl, 10 mM HEPES, 0.1 mM EGTA, 0.3 mM Na-GTP, 1 mM Mg-ATP, and 5 mM phosphocreatine. Adjust the pH to 7.2, and the osmolality to 290 mOsm. Keep the solution in the dark, as ATP and GTP are photosensitive. Prepare 50–100 ml of solution and make 1 ml aliquots. Store the aliquots at −80 °C. Once an aliquot is thawed, it is not recommended to refreeze it or to use it for more than 1 day. After thawing, keep the intracellular solution aliquot on ice and protected from light.

2.3 Coverslips

To obtain optimal results, use the following materials: 12–13 mm glass coverslips, 24-well cell culture plate, 70% EtOH solution, fine forceps (e.g., #55 Dumont), Bunsen burner, sterile DDW, sterile 1× PBS and solutions of adhesion molecules as required by protocol (laminin, polylysine, etc.). Keep the glass coverslips submerged in EtOH until use. Open the 24-well plate inside a clean UV-sterilized laminar-flow hood, and place one single coverslip per well using fine forceps. The EtOH in the coverslips should be removed before placing it in the well, by careful evaporation using a Bunsen burner. Alternatively, after placing coverslips inside the wells, wash the EtOH out by rinsing the coverslips twice with 1 ml of DDW and once with 1 ml of sterile 1× PBS. At this stage, before cell seeding, it is highly recommended to coat glass coverslips with adhesion molecules, such as polylysine/laminin. Apply 0.5 ml of a solution of sterile DDW containing 10 μg/ml poly-D-lysine (cold, from freshly thawed aliquots kept at −20 °C). Let the plate sit for 1–2 h at RT inside a sterile laminar flow hood. Rinse using sterile DDW twice and once more with 1× PBS at RT. Apply

0.2 ml of a solution of sterile 1× PBS containing 20 μg/ml laminin (from freshly thawed aliquots kept at −20 °C). Transfer the plates to 37 °C for at least 4 h (over-night recommended). Finally, wash out the laminin using 1× PBS (rinse twice), before proceeding to cell/neurosphere seeding. If not used immediately, the plates containing polylysine/laminin-coated glass coverslips can be properly wrapped in parafilm and kept at 4 °C for up to 2 weeks (*see* **Note 1**).

2.4 Equipment and Tools

Electrophysiology setup:

Many different types of rigs for electrophysiological recordings exist. The rig that is used for recording from cultured neurons is best suited for recording of activity from neurons derived from stem cells. The following is the system in use by us (*see* Fig. 1) that includes:

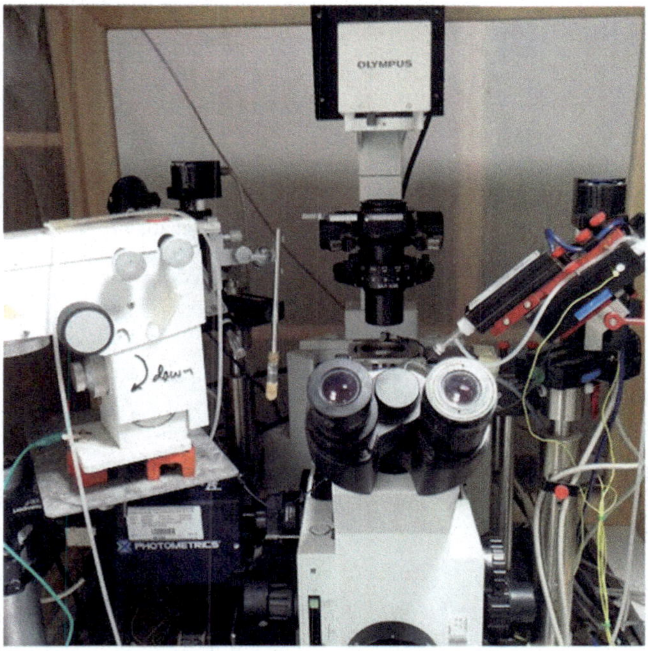

Fig. 1 Electrophysiology setup. An electrophysiological setup for stem cells-derived neurons includes a Faraday cage and an air table housing an inverted microscope (preferably with fluorescent imaging capabilities); an electrode inside a micropipette holder coupled to a manipulator; a recording bath chamber including a ground electrode; and a camera for imaging. Not in the picture: a pipette puller; an amplifier and digitizer; a computer coupled to the system running the recommended software; a perfusion and suction system for solution flow as well as a second manipulator for control of the stage; a manometer; a micropipette holder; disposable syringes, filters, pipettors and tips; an ice bucket. If the microscope is upright instead of inverted, it is recommended to use water submersible objectives. Also, it is highly recommended that the perfusion and suction system are also housed inside the Faraday cage, to reduce interfering noise

1. An inverted Olympus microscope equipped with 40× phase air objective and a low power 10× objective.
2. Semiautomatic controllers that can provide high precision and low drift positioning of micropipettes (Luigs and Neumann Ltd. SM5).
3. The microscope includes high intensity LED light source (Prizmatix Ltd.) for visualizing fluorescent neurons (e.g., following transfection).
4. A Faraday cage and an air table, to reduce electrical noise and mechanical vibrations, respectively.
5. Amplifier for patch-clamp recording is Multiclamp 700B by. Acquisition and analysis software for the experiments are also from Molecular Devices Inc., Clampex 10 and Clampfit 10, respectively.

   Other auxiliary tools include the following:
6. Pipette puller (e.g., model P-87 horizontal puller by Sutter Instruments).
7. Disposable syringes.
8. Disposable 0.2 μm syringe filters.
9. Micropipette holder.
10. Micropipettes (e.g., borosilicate 1.5od glass pipettes by Sutter Instruments).

3 Methods

3.1 Cell Seeding

Differentiated neurons or neural precursor cells can be seeded onto the glass coverslips inside the wells for long periods of time. Coating of coverslips with adhesion molecules should be carried out according to the specific protocol and the desired neuronal identity to be obtained at the end of differentiation. There are two main methods for seeding hESC-derived neurons: through neurosphere aggregates or following cell dissociation.

3.1.1 Neurosphere Aggregates

If this method is chosen, be careful to place a single drop (~20–40 μl) of medium containing neurospheres in the center of the coverslip, after thorough aspiration of any previous liquid. If the neurosphere is seeded in the periphery of the coverslip, recording from these neurons will be much harder. Allow for 1–2 h of seeding and attachment inside the incubator before filling the well with cell medium. Allow at least 48 h for neurons to develop neurite projections (*see* **Note 2**).

3.1.2 Cell Dissociation

If this method is chosen, be careful to use mild dissociating reagents (such as diluted trypsin). Using strong dissociation reagents, or incubating the cells with them for long periods of time, will result in cell death. Eliminate dissociation reagents by gentle centrifugation or by neutralization, when possible. Add 0.9 ml of fresh medium to a single well containing a coverslip at the bottom (use a sterile plastic tip to push sink the coverslip and force air bubbles out). Next, add 0.1 ml of medium containing the dissociated cells, and incubate for 48 h before proceeding to patch-clamp recordings (*see* **Note 3**).

3.2 Pipette Pulling and Filling

1. Pull micropipettes preferably using filamented borosilicate glass, use a pulling protocol that will render micropipettes with a tip diameter of no more than 2 μm (*see* **Note 4**).
2. Use a 1 ml disposable syringe to draw the intracellular solution. Connect to it the filter and the microneedle, and fill the micropipette. For neurons derived from hESCs, usually with small somata, the resistance measured in the bath chamber should be 5–8 MΩ (*see* **Note 5**).
3. If using intracellular dyes, toxins, and drugs inside the pipette, it is best to add them fresh to the intracellular solution before the beginning of recording, and before filtering the solution (*see* **Note 6**).

3.3 Whole-Cell Recording

1. Before removing the coverslip from the well, replace cell incubation medium with filtered extracellular solution (a 20 ml syringe with a filter can be useful). Transfer the coverslip to the recording chamber and fill it with filtered extracellular solution, or start ongoing perfusion.
2. Under the microscope, using visible light and phase contrast microscopy or epifluorescence (e.g., GFP expressing cells), screen the coverslip to identify the neurons selected for recording. Look for cells with clear neuronal morphology. Typical morphology of hESC-derived neurons in-vitro is small round and bright soma, and at least two neurite projections typically protruding from opposite ends of the soma, very thin and long with several arborizing branches (Fig. 2) (*see* **Note 7**).
3. At low magnification, introduce the micropipette into the recording chamber and lower it gradually until approaching the desired cell for recording. Apply constant positive pressure, using a syringe and a manometer. Applying further gentle positive pressure close to the cell can be used to displace debris that can clog the micropipette. Once the micropipette is in position and touching the soma of the cell, apply negative pressure to suck a small part of the cell membrane into the pipette tip. The resistance will increase from 5–8 MΩ (before

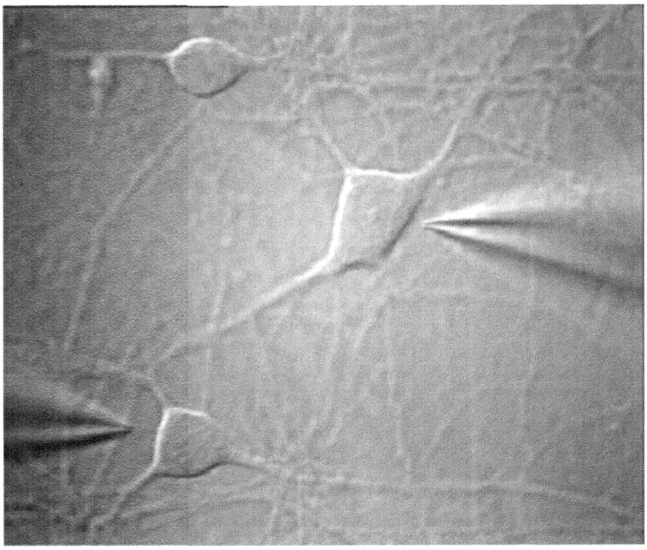

Fig. 2 Morphology of hESC-derived in vitro neurons. Typical morphology of hESC-derived in vitro neurons. Cells present small and round somata, usually brighter than the surroundings as observed using phase-contrast light microscopy. Each neuron typically displays a few growing neurites; their length depends on developmental stage as well as seeding density and post-seeding cell survival. Neurites are usually very thin (~1–2 μm wide), long, and tortuous. In advanced cultures each neurite displays several arborizing subbranches that are even thinner and shorter. In this picture, two separate micropipettes are shown: these could be one for recording and one for puff delivery of drugs and neurotransmitters, or both for simultaneous recording of two cells. Magnification is 40×

touching the cell), to at least 1 GΩ, to achieve a stable membrane seal. At this point, capacitance compensation should be performed.

4. Next, negative pressure should be applied to create a micro-rupture of the membrane, also known as "breaking in." If successful, large but stable capacitance transients will develop. At this point the clamping voltage (usually −60 mV) will be set (*see* **Note 8**).
5. At the end of the recording, the micropipette should be retrieved and disposed. If the recorded cell is to be further analyzed, it is possible to disconnect the micropipette from the cell without disrupting it, by applying gentle positive pressure as the micropipette is slowly moved far away from the cell.

3.4 Pharmacology and Postrecording use of Cell Cultures

1. Homogeneous pharmacological manipulation of all the cells in the culture, can be achieved by dissolving the drug in extracellular solution. Cells can be exposed to the drug by continuous perfusion in and out of the recording chamber, or the drug can

be applied to a static recording chamber that holds a determined amount of extracellular solution for preincubation.

2. Localized pharmacological manipulation can be achieved by using air puffs through a pressure pipette: a micropipette is filled with extracellular solution containing the drug in question, and lowered to a position nearby the cell to be recorded (e.g., ~5–10 μm away, Fig. 2). After successfully braking in and recording from the neuron, the pressure pipette is activated through an external manipulator, which will deliver an air puff on command (*see* **Note 9**).
3. Intracellular pharmacological manipulation can be achieved by dissolving the drug inside the intracellular solution, prior to loading the micropipette. Recordings must start immediately after braking to establish a baseline, before the drug/toxin spreads inside the cell and starts eliciting its effects (*see* **Note 10**).
4. At the end of the recording the coverslip can be removed from the recording chamber and transferred to a chemical hood for fixation with 4% paraformaldehyde (15 min, room temperature, protect from light). Cells can then be used for immunostaining and imaging.

4 Notes

1. Beware that different protocols include different adhesion molecules and/or combinations. The specific composition of the adhesion substrate can significantly alter the outcome of differentiation (i.e., neuronal identity), and should be carefully calibrated for optimal concentration and incubation times.
2. Seeding neurosphere aggregates:

   Pros: as cells are closely packed and developing from a central seeded aggregate, there are higher chances for the formation of synaptic connections.
   Cons: the cells that are suitable for recording will be present in a narrow margin monolayer halo around the central aggregate.
3. Seeding dissociated cells:

   Pros: cells are more evenly spread all across the coverslip, morphology of individual cells can be resolved more easily, and even individual connections between cells can be identified.
   Cons: seeding density must be empirically calibrated, and it will vary according to differentiation protocol, cell line and developmental stage.
4. Protocols for pulling the desired type of micropipette will change according to the puller and the type of glass used. Micropipettes can be fire-polished if needed, to create smooth

edges. The tip of the micropipette should be carefully isolated from any type of contact, as it is extremely fragile.

5. After filling micropipettes with intracellular solution, remove air bubbles by shaking/flicking. Leaving the filled micropipette in a vertical holder for a minute or so, can also help with displacing air bubbles. When introducing the filled micropipette into the extra-cellular solution (inside the recording chamber), apply positive pressure to prevent clogging of the tip.
6. It is recommended to test the intracellular solution's osmolality and pH, especially after adding intracellular dyes, toxins, or drugs.
7. Depending on the differentiation protocol used and the developmental stage of the cells, more complex morphology can be observed and used to identify the cells. Also, in most such cultures, glia cells will also develop. These cells can be easily identified, as they typically show a big, grey, and flat soma with visible nucleus and nucleolus, and with projections that are wide and flat. Recoding from glia cells is harder than from neurons, as they tend to be flat, and these cells do not fire action potentials or participate in fast synaptic communication.
8. After "breaking in," the contents of the intracellular solution will equilibrate with the inner milieu of the cell within minutes. Cells can be recorded from, in either voltage- or current-clamp. Using a "gap-free" recording mode, with a sample rate of 50 μs, at different holding voltages can be used to record spontaneous synaptic events. Recording protocols including several consecutive short steps can be used in voltage-clamp to study intrinsic physiological properties (inward and outward currents), and in current-clamp to explore action potential firing and excitability.
9. The size, strength and duration of the puff needs to be determined and calibrated, in such way that the contents of the pressure pipette will reach the cell, but without damaging it or disrupting the clamp.
10. This approach is useful, especially when the drug in question is membrane impermeant. As the recording micropipette is lowered into the chamber with constant positive pressure, the drug included in the intracellular solution will dilute in the extracellular milieu and reach the cells before the recording begins. Therefore, selection of drugs that are membrane-impermeable is highly recommended.

References

1. Penagarikano O, Mulle JG, Warren ST (2007) The pathophysiology of fragile x syndrome. Annu Rev Genomics Hum Genet 8:109–129
2. Jin P, Warren ST (2000) Understanding the molecular basis of fragile X syndrome. Hum Mol Genet 9:901–908
3. Telias M, Ben-Yosef D (2014) Modeling neurodevelopmental disorders using human pluripotent stem cells. Stem Cell Rev 10:494–511
4. Acab A, Muotri AR (2015) The use of induced pluripotent stem cell technology to advance autism research and treatment. Neurotherapeutics 12:534–545
5. Telias M, Kuznitsov-Yanovsky L, Segal M, Ben-Yosef D (2015) Functional deficiencies in fragile X neurons derived from human embryonic stem cells. J Neurosci 35:15295–15306
6. Telias M, Segal M, Ben-Yosef D (2014) Electrical maturation of neurons derived from human embryonic stem cells. F1000Res 3:196
7. Verkhratsky A, Parpura V (2014) History of electrophysiology and the patch clamp. Methods Mol Biol 1183:1–19
8. Walz W (2007) Patch-clamp analysis advanced techniques. In: Neuromethods, vol 38. 2nd edn. Humana Press, Totowa, NJ, p. x, 475

Chapter 12

Application of Drosophila Model Toward Understanding the Molecular Basis of Fragile X Syndrome

Ha Eun Kong, Junghwa Lim, and Peng Jin

Abstract

Drosophila melanogaster is an ideal model to study Fragile X syndrome (FXS) as it presents us with a toolbox to identify genetic modifiers and to investigate the molecular mechanisms of FXS. Here we describe some of the methods that have been used to study FXS, ranging from reverse genetic screening using the GAL4-UAS system, to mushroom body staining and courtship behavioral assays to examine the learning and memory deficits associated with FXS.

Key words Drosophila genetic screen, Mushroom body staining, Courtship behavioral assay, Fragile X syndrome

1 Introduction

The widely used fruit fly, *Drosophila melanogaster*, is a powerful tool for studying neurodevelopmental disorders, and has been studied for more than a century. Approximately 75% of human disease-causing genes are estimated to be conserved in *D. melanogaster*. Its rapid life cycle, high fecundity, and low-cost maintenance, along with the highly conserved biology, have made the fruit fly a very attractive model to study human disease, and this has contributed to many breakthrough discoveries in biology.

The GAL4-UAS system, first developed by Brand and Perrimon [1] is the most popular tool used in *Drosophila* and has been widely used to perform reverse genetic screens by testing and validating candidate genes for functional effect. Many GAL4 driver lines are available, in which the yeast transcription factor GAL4 is expressed under a cell or tissue-specific promoter such as GMR (Glass Multimer Reporter) for the eye. When these flies are crossed with flies that have GAL4 response elements (UAS) upstream of the desired transgenic element, the resulting progeny express the

Dalit Ben-Yosef and Yoav Mayshar (eds.), *Fragile-X Syndrome: Methods and Protocols*, Methods in Molecular Biology, vol. 1942, https://doi.org/10.1007/978-1-4939-9080-1_12,

transgene in the desired tissues or cells. The Bloomington Drosophila Stock Center and the Vienna Drosophila Research Center, among others, house a large collection of UAS-RNAi knockdown strains that are available to researchers worldwide [2].

The *Drosophila* model system has proven to be especially useful in studying the molecular basis of Fragile X syndrome (FXS). The *dFmr1* gene is the *Drosophila* homologue of the human *FMR1* gene [3]. *dFmr1* behaves similarly to its human counterpart at the molecular level; in fact, *dFmr1* has been shown to regulate the translation of its mRNA targets such as *futsch (Drosophila* ortholog of *MAP1B), chickadee and Rac1* [4–6]. Importantly, flies that lack *dFmr1* demonstrate a clear phenotypic readout: abnormalities in neuromuscular junction (NMJ) synaptic terminals, neural architecture, as well as courtship behavior [3, 5, 7, 8], which point toward learning and memory deficits and are reminiscent of the parallel phenotype seen in human FXS patients. On the other hand, overexpression of *dFmr1* induces apoptosis, which manifest as cell loss in the wing tissue, as well as a severe rough eye phenotype in the flies [3].

We have used the *Drosophila dFmr1* null mutant strains to study the molecular mechanism underlying the altered circadian rhythm behaviors seen in flies and mice lacking FMRP [9]. Furthermore, the rough eye phenotype in flies overexpressing *dFmr1* allowed us to use the fly eye as a tool to uncover the genetic interaction between FMRP and the microRNA pathway [10]. More recently, our group has also used RNAi knockdown of *dFmr1* to show that *dFmr1* triggers a replication stress-induced DNA damage response [11].

In this chapter, we will introduce some of the tools that we have used to study the molecular basis of FXS. To perform the reverse genetic screen to identify the genetic modifiers of FXS, UAS-RNAi knockdown strains against candidate genes can be crossed with flies overexpressing *dFmr1,* that also express GAL4 under the GMR promoter. The enhancement or suppression of the rough eye phenotype can serve as the readout as to whether the candidate gene is a genetic modifier of FXS. The eye phenotype readout can be performed with light microscopy, which should be validated using thin sectioning (*see* Subheading 3.1) [12, 13] and scanning electron microscopy (*see* Subheading 3.2) [14]. The alterations seen in the eye screen can be validated through additional assays covered in this chapter: mushroom body staining to verify the neural architecture (*see* Subheading 3.3) [15], and courtship behavior assay to assess any deficits in learning and memory (*see* Subheading 3.4) [16].

2 Materials

2.1 Thin Sectioning of Adult Drosophila Eyes

1. Reagents.
   - (a) 0.1 M PO_4: 0.2 M Na_2HPO_4, 0.2 M NaH_2PO_4 (*see* **Note 1**).
   - (b) 2% glutaraldehyde (*see* **Note 2**).
   - (c) 2% OsO_4.
   - (d) Ethanol (30%, 50%, 70%, 80%, 90%, and 100%).
   - (e) Propylene oxide.
   - (f) Resin (Durcupan ACM) stored at −80 °C (*see* **Note 3**).
   - (g) DPX Mounting medium.
   - (h) Toluidine solution.
2. Equipment.
   - (a) 1.5 ml microcentrifuge tube.
   - (b) Disposable transfer pipette.
   - (c) Fume hood.
   - (d) Microtome.
   - (e) CO_2.
   - (f) Toothpick.
   - (g) Glass knife boat.
   - (h) Forceps.
   - (i) Aluminum foil.
   - (j) Razor blades.
   - (k) Microscope.
   - (l) Silicone rubber molds.
   - (m) Heating block.
   - (n) Gelatin-coated glass slide.

2.2 Preparation of Drosophila Eye for Scanning Electron Microscopy

1. Reagents.
   - (a) Ethanol (25%, 50%, 75%, and 100%).
   - (b) Hexamethyldisilazane (HMDS).
2. Equipment.
   - (a) Microcentrifuge tubes (1.5 ml).
   - (b) Extended fine tip, large bulb transfer pipette.
   - (c) Aluminum specimen mount (15 × 10 mm cylinders) (Ted Pella Inc.).
   - (d) Double-stick carbon conductive tabs (ϕ12 mm).
   - (e) Fume hood.

2.3 Mushroom Body Staining

1. Reagent.
   (a) Fixative solution: 4% paraformaldehyde in PBS, 40 mM Lysine, pH 7.2 (*see* **Note 4**).
   (b) 1× PBS (pH 7.2).
   (c) 1× PBHT: 20 mM PO_4, 0.5 M NaCl, 0.2% Triton X-100, pH 7.4 (*see* **Note 5**).
   (d) Blocking solution: 5% Normal Goat Serum in 1× PBHT.
   (e) 0.12 M Tris–HCl (pH 7.2).
   (f) 95% ethanol.
   (g) Vectashield medium (Vector Labs)
   (h) Primary antibody: Anti-fasciclin II (DSHB).
   (i) Secondary antibody: Anti-mouse IgG antibody conjugated with Alexa 488 (Invitrogen).
2. Equipment.
   (a) 9-well pyrex spot plate.
   (b) A pair of Dumont #5 forceps.
   (c) Pipette and pipette tips.
   (d) Microcentrifuge tube (1.5 ml).
   (e) 3D Rocker.
   (f) Dissection microscope.
   (g) Disposable petri dish (diameter 140 mm).
   (h) Aluminum foil.
   (i) Gelatin-coated glass slide.
   (j) Microscope cover glasses.
   (k) Nail polish.
   (l) Disposable petri dish (diameter 47 mm).
   (m) Fine soft brush.
   (n) Glass depression slide.

2.4 Courtship Behavior Assay

1. Reagents.
   (a) CO_2.
   (b) *Drosophila melanogaster*.
   (c) Food media.
   (d) Distilled water.
2. Equipment.
   (a) Aspirator.
      - LDPE Quick Connector Fittings.
      - 3/16ID & 5/16OD silicone tubing.
      - Fine mesh cloth.

(b) Courtship chamber.
   - Size 8 × 8 × 5 mm^3 (*see* **Note 6**).

(c) Filter paper: Whatman 3MM Chromatography Paper.

(d) Incubator (see **Note 7**).

(e) White light: for setting up inside incubator.

(f) Video recording system.
   - High-resolution camera.
   - Computer: connected to camera.
   - Stand.

(g) Graduated Transport Tubes (5 ml).

(h) Vials.

(i) Cotton ball.

3 Methods

3.1 Thin Sectioning of Adult Drosophila Eyes

Gloves should be worn throughout to protect from toxicity. Due to the toxicity of the resin, the benchtop and all contact surfaces must be covered with aluminum foil. Following the procedure, all waste including the aluminum should be baked at 70 °C before discarding.

3.1.1 Fly Head Dissection

1. Dissect fly head with forceps and carefully cut off one of the eyes with new razor blade to help penetration of the fixative solution.
2. Place the dissected head into 2% glutaraldehyde in 0.1 M PO_4 on ice.

   Do not keep the dissected heads in fixative solution for longer than 15 min.
3. Spin down in the centrifuge for a few seconds to submerge the fly heads.
4. In the fume hood, add an equal volume of 2% OsO_4 in 0.1 M PO_4 and incubate for 30 min on ice.
5. Remove glutaraldehyde–OsO_4 mixture and replace with cold 0.1 M PO_4 buffer by filling the tube for washing.
6. Discard the phosphate buffer and add 0.5 ml of fresh 2% OsO_4 in 0.1 M PO_4 to the dissected head. Incubate for 1–6 h on ice (*see* **Note 8**).

3.1.2 Dehydration

1. By using a disposable transfer pipette, discard the Osmium solution into the proper waste bottle, and add 1 ml 30% ethanol. Then incubate for 10 min on ice.

2. Repeat the step above with 50%, 70%, 80%, 90%, and 100% ethanol.
3. Incubate with 100% ethanol for 10 min at room temperature twice.

3.1.3 Embedding

1. Take aliquots of resin out from −80 °C and place in the 37–42 °C water bath.
2. Replace the ethanol with 1 ml propylene oxide in the fume hood, and incubate for 10 min at room temperature.
3. Repeat propylene oxide wash twice.
4. Leave 0.5 ml propylene oxide, add 0.5 ml Durcupan resin to the propylene oxide, and mix well by using disposable transfer pipette. When the fly head is mixed with propylene oxide–resin mixture, allow each head to be covered with the mixture by using the transfer pipette to pipette up and down carefully.
5. Incubate overnight at room temperature.
6. Replace the propylene oxide–resin mixture with pure resin, and mix well with sunk heads by pipetting. Incubate the heads in the resin for at least 4 h at room temperature (*see* **Note 9**).
7. Pick the heads up from the resin tube one at a time, and place each head in an edge of each well of the rubber mold (Fig. 1). The head should be placed with the anterior up and the eye to be sectioned should be close to the front mold wall. Each well of the mold is numbered so you can keep track of your samples. Make sure to record the number of the mold for each sample.
8. Fill each mold with pure resin, making sure that the head is aligned correctly again using a needle or sharp toothpick.

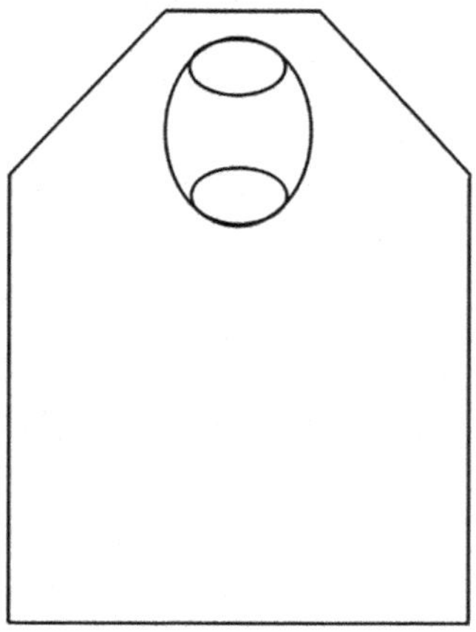

Fig. 1 Embedding the fly in the resin. Put a drop of resin at the edge of mold and then place a fly head in the resin. The head should be placed anterior up and the eye to be sectioned is to be close to the front mold wall. Fill each mold with pure resin, align the head correctly again using needle of toothpick

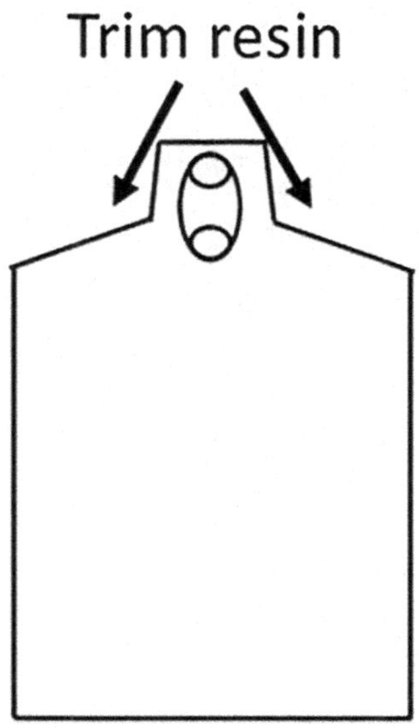

Fig. 2 Trimming the resin. Cut away resin around the head to make a trapezoid

9. Bake the molds overnight at 70 °C with all the toxic waste that was in contact with the resin, including the aluminum waste that was used to cover surfaces. After baking, the resin is no longer toxic.

3.1.4 Sectioning

1. Take the block off from mold, use a chuck for microtome, and set the block up to trim. The eye should be placed up in the chuck (Fig. 2).
2. Cut away resin around the head to make a trapezoid form so that the eye is placed inside the form with razor blade under the dissection microscope.
3. Mount the trimmed block in the microtome.
4. Start to cut sections to 1 μm and the actual surface of head will be exposed.
5. Transfer 10–20 actual head sections to a drop of water on a gelatin coated glass slide by using a very fine brush (*see* **Note 10**).
6. Place the slide with collected sections on a heating block (70–80 °C) and wait until water has evaporated and the sections stick to the slide.
7. Cover the section with several drops toluidine solution, and place the slide on a heating plate for 1 min.
8. Wash the slide with water and dry completely. Mount with DPX mounting medium.

3.2 Preparation of Drosophila Eye for Scanning Electron Microscopy

1. Anesthetize the adult flies with CO_2.
2. Place ten flies into 1.5 ml centrifuge tubes containing 1 ml of 25% ethanol and incubate for 12–24 h at RT.
3. Discard the 25% ethanol with an extended fine tip transfer pipette, and replace with the 1 ml of 50% ethanol (handle with care to keep the fly eyes intact, and be careful not to disturb the eyes) and incubate for 12–24 h at RT.
4. Discard the 50% ethanol with an extended fine tip transfer pipette and replace with the 1 ml of 75% ethanol (handle with care to keep the fly eyes intact) and incubate for 12–24 h at RT.
5. Repeat **step 4** with 75% ethanol.
6. Repeat **step 5** with 100% ethanol (*see* **Note 11**).
7. Discard the 100% ethanol and replace with 500 μl of hexamethyldisilazane (HMDS) and incubate for 3 min in fume hood.
8. Discard the HMDS and replace with 500 μl of HMDS again, and incubate for 1–2 h in fume hood.
9. Remove all HMDS and dry in fume hood overnight, keeping the cap open.
10. Place the carbon conductive tab on specimen cylinder.
11. Cut off the all legs and wings of the prepared flies and mount flies on the tabs of specimen (*see* **Note 12**). The prepared samples can be stored limitlessly in vacuum desiccator.

3.3 Whole Mount Brain Immunostaining (Mushroom Body Staining)

3.3.1 Sample Preparation

1. Prepare a small petri dish (47 mm diameter) with 95% ethanol, and soak flies for 30–60 s. Do not leave the flies soaking over 1 min.
2. Pick the flies up from the ethanol with brush, and keep flies in PBS until ready to be dissected.
3. Brain dissection: dissect fly brain in depression slide with PBS.
4. After dissection, rinse brain in PBS to clean up tissue debris.
5. Fixation: fix the brain in 4% paraformaldehyde in PBS with Lysine for 20 min at room temperature (RT) and/or can be extended up to 3 h on 4 °C. Do not exceed the time limit for fixation.
6. After fixation, rinse brain in PBS to clean up the paraformaldehyde.
7. Wash in 1× PBHT for 10 min on 3D rocker twice. Always remove old buffer with pipette and replace with fresh buffer immediately. Do not let brain dry. Starting from the washing step, all steps should be performed with the 3D rocker to ensure good mixing.

3.3.2 Immunostaining

1. Penetration: remove the washing buffer, and replace with 1% PBHT for 1 h. Keep the 9-well spot plate in a 140 mm petri dish lined with a wet paper towel to prevent drying out during long incubations. Cover the lid.
2. Blocking: Remove 1% PBHT solution, and replace with 5% normal goat serum for 2 h at room temperature (*see* **Note 13**).
3. Primary antibody incubation: prepare anti-fasciclin II (DSHB) dilution (1:1000) with 5% blocking solution in microcentrifuge tube. Discard blocking solution, add 200–300 μl of primary antibody, and incubate overnight at 4 °C.
4. Washing: Remove the primary antibody, wash with 1× PBHT buffer solution for 20 min three times (*see* **Note 14**).
5. Secondary antibody incubation: Dilute anti-mouse IgG antibody conjugated with Alexa 488 (1:1000, Invitrogen, Carlsbad, CA) with 5% NGS blocking solution. Discard the washing buffer, add 200–300 μl of secondary antibody, and incubate for 2 h at room temperature, covered with aluminum foil.
6. Washing: Remove the secondary antibody, wash with 1× PBHT buffer solution for 20 min three times, and follow washes by 0.12 M Tris–HCl for 10 min three times.
7. Mounting: Transfer the brains to gelatin coated glass slide by pipetting with solution (*see* **Note 15**). Remove the solution on the slide without touching the brain, drop a drop of Vectashield medium (Vectar Lab), and cover with microscope coverslip without bubbles. Seal the coverslip with nail polish.

3.4 Courtship Behavior Assay

3.4.1 Preparing Equipment

1. Making a mouth aspirator.
   - (a) Cut silicone tube to 15–18 in.
   - (b) Insert an LDPE Quick Connector female to one side of silicone tube.
   - (c) Insert an LDPE Quick Connector male with fine mesh cloth to other side of tube.
2. Construct incubator.
   - (a) Install the camera considering height and focus.
   - (b) Connect camera with computer for observation and check that it records well.
   - (c) Set up bright white light.
   - (d) Maintain 50% relative humidity.

3.4.2 Preparing Adult Flies

Unless testing for differences in aging, use 4–5-day-old females and males in the experiments.

1. Rear flies on a standard cornmeal/agar medium at 25 °C with a light–dark (12 h-L–12 h-D) cycle and under 50% relative humidity.

2. Collect male flies under CO_2 within 12–18 h after eclosion and house individually in a food vial for 3–4 days (*see* **Note 16**).
3. Collect virgin *CS* (Canton-S) females within 12 h after eclosion and house them together in a food vial. Confirm virginity by confirming the absence of progeny in the food vial. Keep 10–15 females in each vial.
4. Prepare mated *CS* females by housing a single virgin female with 3–4 mature *CS* males for 18–24 h in a small vial containing food and then use them for conditioning (*see* **Note 17**).
5. Decapitate virgin *CS* females 10 min before use with fine scissors under CO_2 and use only moving flies within 1 h.

3.4.3 Basal Courtship Assay

1. Set up the courtship chamber ($8 \times 8 \times 5$ mm^3).
2. Cut the filter paper in a circle (diameter 8 mm) while wearing gloves.
3. Place the filter paper at the bottom of each courtship chamber and add 15 μl of double distilled water just before the experiment. Label each chamber with the fly identification number and date.
4. Transfer the tester male to a chamber by aspiration and acclimate for 10 min.
5. Introduce a single courtee (i.e., intact or decapitated virgin *CS* female) with an aspirator.
6. Place the courtship chamber in the incubator under the camera, and record for 1 h.
7. Score the individual courtship steps in the first 10 min of the video: That is, orientation and following, tapping, singing, licking, attempted copulation, and copulation [17].
8. Analyze the data.

3.4.4 Conditioned Courtship Assay

1. Set up the courtship chamber ($8 \times 8 \times 5$ mm^3).
2. Cut the filter paper in a circle (diameter 8 mm).
3. Place the filter paper at the bottom of each courtship chamber and add 15 μl of double distilled water just before the experiment. Ensure to label each chamber with the fly identification number and date.
4. Transfer a tester male to a chamber by aspiration and acclimate for 10 min.
5. Introduce a single mated CS female with aspirator.
6. Place the courtship chamber in the incubator under camera, and record for 1 h (Training phase).
7. For control, transfer a single male and keep it alone for 1 h in the incubator. You do not need to record it (Mock exposure).

8. For the acquisition test, after 1 h of training, transfer the trained male into other new chamber and introduce the decapitated female virgin CS.
9. Record for 20 min and score the individual steps in the first 10 min of the video.
10. To test short term memory (e.g., 1 h, 3 h), after 1 h training, transfer the trained male to the food vial individually again and keep it in the incubator for a short term (e.g., 1 h, 3 h).
11. Prepare a new courtship chamber with the decapitated female virgin CS, transfer the trained male in the chamber, and record for 20 min.
12. Score individual steps in the first 10 min of the video, and analyze.
13. Perform the same test with the mock exposure male.

4 Notes

1. A 0.1 M PO_4 is made by mixing 0.2 M Na_2HPO_4 and 0.2 M NaH_2PO_4 in a 72:28 ratio, and add an equal volume of double distilled water (e.g., 72 ml of 0.2 M Na_2HPO_4 + 28 ml of 0.2 M NaH_2PO_4 + 100 ml of water will make 200 ml of the buffer). Keep the solution on ice.
2. Prepare 2% glutaraldehyde in 0.1 M PO_4 and aliquot 200ul in 1.5 ml tubes for each sample on ice.
3. Follow the Cold Spring Harbor protocol to prepare the resin [18].
4. Make a fresh solution for every experiment. In a beaker add 1× PBS 90 ml, paraformaldehyde 4 g. Heat with stirring until just dissolved. Make sure not to boil the solution. Cool down the solution on ice and then add 2 ml of 2 M lysine 2 ml. Mix and adjust with 1× PBS buffer solution to 100 ml with graduated cylinder. After making 100 ml of paraformaldehyde solution, aliquot by 1 ml, and store at −80 °C.
5. First, make the stock solution: 5× PBHS (5×, 0.2 M PO4, 5 M NaCl, pH 7.4). In a 1 l beaker, add sodium phosphate monobasic ($NaH_2PO_4 \cdot H_2O$) 13.8 g, sodium chloride (NaCl) 146.1 g, and 800 ml of double distilled water. Mix well with magnetic stir bar on the plate until all components are dissolved. Adjust pH to 7.4 with NaOH and HCl solution. Transfer to a 1 l graduated cylinder, and adjust to 1 l with double distilled water. Filter with disposable filter unit, and store at room temperature. To make 1× PBHT, in a 1 l beaker add 200 ml of 5× PBHS, 2 ml of Triton X-100, around 700 ml of

double distilled water, and mix well with a magnetic stir bar at a low speed, without bubbles. Transfer everything to a 1 l graduated cylinder and adjust to 1 l with double distilled water.

6. The courtship chamber should be cleaned with ethanol and then rinsed with distilled water several times to remove residual fly scents. After rinse, it should be left to dry by air.
7. The incubator should be controlled in temperature and humidity relatively. The temperature should be kept at 25 °C and the humidity should be maintained 50% relatively with a light–dark cycle.
8. Leave on ice overnight.
9. Incubate overnight at room temperature.
10. A very fine brush is necessary to be able to pick up the very thin sections. You can make your own fine brush by attaching one strand of very fine brush hair to a toothpick using nail polish.
11. Once in 100% ethanol, the exterior morphology of the fly eye is stable for at least 1 month.
12. The heads of the flies should be arranged outward and parallel with the tab in order to reduce spending time in orienting the samples.
13. Can keep overnight or several days at 4 °C, making sure that it does not dry out.
14. Can first wash for 20 min, keep the second washing solution for overnight at 4 °C, and perform the last wash for 20 min at room temperature. It depends on the signal and background condition of samples.
15. The pipette tip wall should be wet inside before pipetting to prevent the brain being stuck in the tip.
16. Prepare test tubes for collecting males and keep them individually; each 5 ml test tube should be filled with 1.8 ml standard cornmeal/agar medium, and covered with small pieces of cotton ball. Keeping the males separate ensures that the males avoid social experience that might affect their behavior.
17. Prepare the mated female the day before the experiment. Before use, pick out one female and check the genitalia or check if the female has laid egg on food vial to verify that mating has taken place.

References

1. Brand AH, Perrimon N (1993) Targeted gene expression as a means of altering cell fates and generating dominant phenotypes. Development 118:401–415
2. Dietzl G, Chen D, Schnorrer F et al (2007) A genome-wide transgenic RNAi library for conditional gene inactivation in drosophila. Nature 448:151–156

3. Wan L, Dockendorff TC, Jongens TA et al (2000) Characterization of dFMR1, a Drosophila melanogaster homolog of the fragile X mental retardation protein. Mol Cell Biol 20:8536–8547
4. Lee A, Li W, Xu K et al (2003) Control of dendritic development by the Drosophila fragile X-related gene involves the small GTPase Rac1. Development 130:5543–5552
5. Zhang YQ, Bailey AM, Matthies HJ et al (2001) Drosophila fragile X-related gene regulates the MAP1B homolog Futsch to control synaptic structure and function. Cell 107:591–603
6. Tessier CR, Broadie K (2008) Drosophila fragile X mental retardation protein developmentally regulates activity-dependent axon pruning. Development 135:1547–1557
7. Morales J, Hiesinger PR, Schroeder AJ et al (2002) Drosophila fragile X protein, DFXR, regulates neuronal morphology and function in the brain. Neuron 34:961–972
8. Dockendorff TC, Su HS, McBride SMJ et al (2002) Drosophila lacking dfmr1 activity show defects in circadian output and fail to maintain courtship interest. Neuron 34:973–984
9. Xu S, Poidevin M, Han E et al (2012) Circadian rhythm-dependent alterations of gene expression in drosophila brain lacking fragile X mental retardation protein. PLoS One 7: e37937
10. Jin P, Zarnescu DC, Ceman S et al (2004) Biochemical and genetic interaction between the fragile X mental retardation protein and the microRNA pathway. Nat Neurosci 7:113–117
11. Zhang W, Cheng Y, Li Y et al (2014) A feed-forward mechanism involving Drosophila fragile X mental retardation protein triggers a replication stress-induced DNA damage response. Hum Mol Genet 23:5188–5196
12. Jenny A (2011) Preparation of adult drosophila eyes for thin sectioning and microscopic analysis. J Vis Exp 54:2959
13. Rubin L (1990) Rubin Lab Manual, 2nd edition. http://jfly.iam.utokyo.ac.jp/html/manuals/pdf/Rubin_Lab_Manual90.pdf
14. Wolff T (2011) Preparation of drosophila eye specimens for scanning electron microscopy. Cold Spring Harb. Protoc. 2011, 11:1383–1385. https://doi.org/10.1101/pdb.prot066506
15. Helfrich-Förster C (2007) Immunohistochemistry in Drosophila. In: Rosato E. (eds) Circadian Rhythms. Methods in Molecular Biology™, vol 362. Humana Press
16. Lim J, Fernandez AI, Hinojos SJ et al (2017) The mushroom body D1 dopamine receptor controls innate courtship drive. Genes Brain Behav 17(2):158–167
17. Yamamoto D, Koganezawa M (2013) Genes and circuits of courtship behaviour in drosophila males. Nat Rev Neurosci 14:681–692
18. (2011) Durcupan resin. Cold Spring Harb Protoc 2011:pdb.rec12381

Chapter 13

Fragile X Syndrome Pre-Clinical Research: Comparing Mouse- and Human-Based Models

Michael Telias

Abstract

Despite almost 30 years of biomedical research, a treatment or cure for fragile X syndrome (FXS) is not yet available. The reasons behind this are varied, and among them are discrepancies in both research methodologies and research models. For many years, the *fmr1* knockout mouse model dominated the field, and was used to draw important conclusions. The establishment of FXS-human cellular models called these conclusions into question, showing conflicting evidence. Discrepancies in FXS research, between mouse and human, might arise from differences inherent to each species, and from the use of different methodologies. This chapter summarizes these discrepancies and evaluates their impact on the current status of clinical trials.

Key words FXS pharmacology, FXS treatment, FXS cure, Clinical trials, Clinical trials in FXS, Neurodevelopmental disorders, Treatment of neurodevelopmental disorders

1 Introduction: A Brief History of FXS Research

In 1991, Verkerk et al. identified the human FMR1 gene for the first time, showing that lack of FMR1 expression was the cause behind FXS [1]. Initially, both human and mouse tissues were used to study the expression and function of FMR1 and FMRP [2, 3]. Upon the introduction of the *fmr1* knockout mouse ($fmr1^{-/-}$) in 1994, this model became the most dominant in the field for the next 20 years [4]. The $fmr1^{-/-}$ mouse was used to uncover an abundance of data regarding the molecular and cellular functions of Fmrp. Systematic comparison of human and murine FXS cells was still carried out, but the reproducibility of these results was strongly limited due to the restricted availability of postmortem human nervous tissue samples, and their wide heterogeneity [5]. As compared to sporadic, ad hoc human tissue samples, the transgenic mouse is a much more reliable model. Therefore, most hypotheses proposed to explain the molecular mechanisms responsible for FXS neuropathology were drawn from data

Dalit Ben-Yosef and Yoav Mayshar (eds.), *Fragile-X Syndrome: Methods and Protocols*, Methods in Molecular Biology, vol. 1942,
https://doi.org/10.1007/978-1-4939-9080-1_13,

obtained using *fmr1*$^{-/-}$ mice. Based on these hypotheses, researchers and clinicians designed clinical trials meant to cure or ameliorate disorders and symptoms associated with FXS. Unfortunately, so far, all of these clinical trials have failed. One of the reasons for this failure might be the inability to validate the results obtained in *fmr1*$^{-/-}$ mice in comparable human-based models.

In 2007, Eiges et al. published a seminal article describing the molecular and cellular phenotype of a human embryonic stem cell line carrying the full FMR1 mutation (FX-hESC) [6]. Later on, with the generation of the first human induced pluripotent stem cells (hiPSCs) through reprogramming [7], the field of disease modeling using stem cells grew rapidly, and it was subsequently applied to FXS research [8, 9]. Human pluripotent cells (i.e., hESCs and hiPSCs) offer a means to validate hypotheses obtained in animal models, and furthermore uncover new insights into FXS pathophysiology that might be present only in human cells. While cells growing in-vitro are not a whole organism, and lack the complexity of tissue layering and systemic cellular communication, recent developments such as the induction of organoids that resemble miniature human brains [10] could make the case that the future of FXS research lies with methodologies based on FX-hESC and FX-hiPSC, rather than on mice.

2 Pros and Cons of Mouse Versus Human FXS Models

When discussing the advantages and disadvantages of each research model in FXS, we should discriminate between intrinsic methodological differences vs. FXS-specific features [11, 12]. For example, regardless of the disease being studied, neuronal circuitry between brain areas cannot be explored in stem cells-derived neurons differentiated in-vitro. Table 1a summarizes the most important intrinsic methodological discrepancies between mouse and human stem cells as research platforms, while Table 1b includes major discrepancies specific for FXS.

The first and most important difference between *fmr1*$^{-/-}$ animals and FX-hESCs/hiPSCs lies within the FMR1 mutation itself [13]. In humans, the expansion of the CGG-rich region upstream to the FMR1 promoter to more than 200 repeats, results in abnormal patterns of gene and protein expression during the first months of embryonic development. Only later in embryonic life, a hypermethylation event completely silences FMR1 transcription. In contrast, animals do not show CGG-repeat expansion, and every *fmr1*$^{-/-}$ mouse is the product of genomic manipulation. These animals do not express *fmr1* in any cell, and their whole development takes place in the absence of Fmrp. In other words, while humans experience a developmentally regulated inactivation of FMR1, animals do not. Moreover, since FMR1 is located in the X

Table 1a
Main differences in research methodology between mouse and hESCs/hiPSCs

	Mouse	hESCs	hiPSCs
Research modality	Whole-organism, in-vivo, ex-vivo, in-vitro (i.e., primary cultures, mESCs)	In-vitro; cells can be grafted in animal hosts; can be induced to create organoids ("mini-brains")	
Source	Wild-type/transgenic lab mice	Human blastocytes carrying mutations	Patient's biopsy
Management	Mouse colony management: 21 days gestation period, weaning, selective breeding, euthanasia procedures	Cell culture management: frequent passages, accumulation of random mutations, tissue priming for specific lineages, media, growth factors	
Genetic background	Individuals virtually identical to each other due to inbreeding	Variability like that found in the human population. Can be used to create isogenic cell lines with identical genetic background	
Development	In-utero	In-vitro directed neuronal differentiation.	
Behavior & anatomy	Available behavioral tests (limited comparison to human subjects). Easy identification of anatomical organization	Impossible	
Electrophysiology	Advanced: patch-clamp, field potentials, MEA, EEG, MRI	Limited: mostly patch-clamp, MEA possible	
Gene manipulation	Difficult: conditional KO, in-utero electroporation, in situ vs. systemic viral transduction	Easy: transfection, electroporation, viral transduction, CRISPR	

chromosome, its differential inactivation causes significant phenotypic differences between male and female human patients, due to imprinting and female mosaicism. However, in the mouse, both males and females are complete knockouts, leading to similar phenotype between the sexes. At an even more fundamental level, it still remains largely unknown whether FMRP's RNA and protein targets in human neurons coincide with those in mouse neurons, and whether molecular targets of FMRP binding and activity change depending on specific neuronal identity. For example, the most extensive study on mRNA targets of FMRP was conducted on human cell culture, mouse ovaries and human brain [14].

On the other end of the spectrum, in spite of these profound differences between mouse and human, the mouse model still

Table 1b
FXS-specific differences between research strategies

	fmr1$^{-/-}$ mouse	FX-hESCs	FX-hiPSCs
FMR1 mutation	Point mutation (incidence in humans is 1%)	>200 CGG repeats (incidence in humans is 99%)	
XY vs XX	Similar phenotype	Different phenotype	
FMR1 silencing	Does not mimic the disease in humans: no expression at any developmental stage, no hypermethylation event	Mimics the disease in humans: expression in undifferentiated cultures, methylation-dependent silencing upon induction of differentiation	Mixed: reprogrammed from methylated tissues, reactivation may occur in some clones/lines
RNA toxicity	Probably never happens	Possibly part of the mechanism behind phenotypic abnormalities	Hard to determine, depends on methylation status after reprogramming
FMRP targets	Partial overlap between mouse and human targets of FMRP (evolutionary distance)	Full overlap. Targets may change by cell types or developmental stage	
Experimental controls	Age-matched nonmutated mice from the same strain	Non-FMR1-mutated hESC lines	Biopsy from healthy siblings/relatives

Abbreviations for Tables 1a and 1b: *mESCs* - mouse embryonic stem cells, *hESCs* - human embryonic stem cells, *hiPSCs* - human induced pluripotent stem cells; *PGD* - preimplantation genetic diagnosis, *MEA* - multielectrode array, *EEG* - electroencephalogram, *MRI* - magnetic resonance imaging, *KO* - knockout

offers a methodological range much larger than human pluripotent cells. Anatomical and behavioral aspects of FXS cannot be explored using FX-hESCs or FX-hiPSCs, for obvious reasons. In this sense, with the exception of human patients themselves, the *fmr1*$^{-/-}$ model has no alternative. However, how well the *fmr1*$^{-/-}$ recapitulates the social anxiety and sensory overload of FXS patients is open to debate. For example, 20–25% of teenagers with FXS will suffer from spontaneous and temporary epilepsy. In contrast, in 100% of *fmr1*$^{-/-}$ mice, it is possible to elicit epileptic-like seizures using loud noises at all stages of life. However, many other knockout mouse strains, in which *fmr1* remains unchanged, also exhibit similar audiogenic epileptic convulsions, calling into question the use of seizure induction as a reliable test to analyze FXS-associated symptoms [15]. In addition, while human FXS patients show increased levels of anxiety and hyperactivity, *fmr1*$^{-/-}$ mice were shown to be hyperactive like humans, but display reduced anxiety-like behaviors, as compared to control mice [12].

In summary, mice have many methodological advantages as compared to hESCs/hiPSCs in studying molecular aspects of the disease, but FX-hESCs/hiPSCs are important for investigating key aspects of FXS pathology that are problematic in *fmr1*$^{-/-}$ mice. While no research model is perfect, and all are approximations of the real thing, knowing the intricate differences between the main models can help researchers decide which one will be more suitable for a specific set of questions.

3 Leading Hypotheses, Conflicting Evidence, and Clinical Trials

Hypotheses explaining natural phenomena are always based on experimental evidence. The limitations of a specific research model will significantly impact the results obtained, therefore affecting the formulation of hypotheses. In the field of FXS research, the most widespread hypotheses, were drawn exclusively from data obtained using *fmr1*$^{-/-}$ mice and were not confirmed on a human-based research model, before entering clinical trials, that unfortunately all failed. On the other hand, human validation can be technically difficult, and in some cases, ethically impossible. New research models need to be created to circumvent these issues, but there is no doubt that our field suffers from *fmr1*$^{-/-}$ mouse chauvinism and confirmation bias.

The first proposed mechanism to explain the intellectual deficits of FXS was developed based on *fmr1*$^{-/-}$ mice [16, 17]. This hypothesis, known as "the mGluR theory of FXS," states that loss of Fmrp in the *fmr1*$^{-/-}$ mouse results in a pathological increase in synaptic signaling through metabotropic glutamate receptors (mGluRs), resulting in increased long-term depression (LTD), purportedly explaining cognitive deficiencies in FXS patients. Since then, studies on *fmr1*$^{-/-}$ mice by other labs, have shown that Fmrp absence affects intrinsic properties of the presynaptic side as well [18]. More importantly, no study has shown validation of the "mGluR theory" in any human-based model [19]. When we analyzed the electrophysiological properties of FX human neurons derived from FX-hESCs, we found evidence for both presynaptic and postsynaptic deficiencies, and no evidence whatsoever for the involvement of enhanced mGluRs-mediated signaling in human FX-synapses [20].

Another hypothesis of FXS pathology was built around robust evidence obtained in *fmr1*$^{-/-}$ mice, indicating that several brain areas display significantly increased levels of glycogen synthase kinase 3 beta (Gsk-3β) protein [21]. In humans like in mice, GSK-3β plays pivotal roles in development and homeostasis, serving as a checkpoint at which many different intracellular pathways intersect each other. As such, the discovery that GSK-3β is involved in the pathophysiology of FXS in humans could have importance consequences on potential treatments. Indeed, when *fmr1*$^{-/-}$ mice were treated with Gsk-3β inhibitors, symptoms were effectively rescued [22].However, in this case too, no human validation of this observation has been reported so far. Moreover, we have previously demonstrated that in FX human neural precursor cells derived from hESCs, a partial decrease in FMR1 expression was associated with a decrease in GSK-3β levels, opposite to the results obtained in mouse [23]. Furthermore, inhibiting FMR1 expression in control cells reduced GSK-3β levels, overexpression of FMR1 in FX-cells increased GSK-3β, and none of these manipulations had any significant effect on β-catenin, the main molecular target of GSK-3β. These results indicate, at the very least, that the GSK-3β hypothesis of FXS pathology might be less relevant for FX human patients.

Last but not least, a GABA hypothesis of FXS pathology was also backed by an important body of evidence obtained from the *fmr1*$^{-/-}$ mouse [24]. According to this hypothesis, both ionotropic (GABA-A) and metabotropic (GABA-B) receptors are involved in FXS pathophysiology. GABA-A mediated signaling is associated with FXS during early development of the central nervous system, during which GABA-A receptors are key players in an excitatory-to-inhibitory developmental switch that is delayed in *fmr1*$^{-/-}$ mice [25]. This is a fascinating hypothesis, but translating it into a feasible treatment for FXS could prove difficult or even impossible to achieve, as this developmental switch occurs in-utero. Regarding GABA-B receptors, it has been shown that their expression is reduced in the forebrain of adult *fmr1*$^{-/-}$ mice [26]. At the presynaptic terminal, GABA-B receptors reduce the amount of glutamate released into the synaptic cleft, therefore preventing hyperexcitation. According to this, hyperexcitability in FXS is caused by decreased GABA-B-mediated attenuation of glutamate secretion. However, as mentioned before, no validation in human has been provided for this hypothesis, and therefore whether this is true in humans remains to be shown. In addition, data from human FX neurons derived from FX-hESCs, contradicts some of the findings in mice [27]. While we observed a pronounced difference in GABA-A mediated responses and receptor subunits expression in human FX neurons as compared to nonmutated controls, there was no evidence for the involvement of GABA-B.

Based on these three hypotheses, and others not mentioned here, patients were recruited for several clinical trials [11]. Based on the "mGluR theory," patients were given Mavoglurant (a mGluR antagonist) or Ampalex (an AMPA allosteric modulator; clinical trial IDs NCT01253629 and NCT00054730, respectively). Since GSK-3β is inhibited by lithium, the findings in *fmr1*$^{-/-}$ mice were used in clinical trials aimed to treat FXS patients with Lithium, an FDA-approved drug currently in use for several psychiatric disorders. The possible involvement of GABA-B receptors in FXS pathology was also provided as a reason to engage patients in clinical trials, testing the effects of Arbaclofen, a GABA-B agonist (NCT01013480). However, none of these trials have succeeded in promoting the development of treatments for FXS patients. It is therefore important that all findings from mice studies will be validated on human in-vitro research models, and that such validation will eventually become a standard procedure in preclinical studies.

4 Future Approaches

Modern medical sciences must evolve beyond this "mouse-to-clinic" approach when dealing with complex neurodevelopmental disorders, such as FXS and Autism. The idea that one single cellular component, such as a single receptor or enzyme, is responsible for the plethora of behavioral disorders and cognitive impairments associated with FXS is, perhaps, naïve. New approaches to investigate and to treat need to emerge. For example, in the future it might be feasible to replace defective (i.e., FMR1-mutated) adult neural stem cells that reside in the subventricular zone, with a graft of autologous reprogrammed stem cells in which the mutation has been corrected [28], repopulating the brain with FMRP-expressing neurons (cell therapy). In the far future, with the advent of CRISPR-related technologies applied to human embryos or even adults, it will be possible to physically remove the CGG-repeat expansion from the FMR1 locus, resetting its methylation status through genomic therapy, currently available only in-vitro [29–31]. However, until then, it is imperative that FXS researchers validate their animal-based findings in human models, taking into account the pros and cons intrinsic to every model and system.

References

1. Verkerk AJ et al (1991) Identification of a gene (FMR-1) containing a CGG repeat coincident with a breakpoint cluster region exhibiting length variation in fragile X syndrome. Cell 65 (5):905–914
2. Hinds HL et al (1993) Tissue specific expression of FMR-1 provides evidence for a functional role in fragile X syndrome. Nat Genet 3 (1):36–43
3. Abitbol M et al (1993) Nucleus basalis magnocellularis and hippocampus are the major sites of FMR-1 expression in the human fetal brain. Nat Genet 4(2):147–153
4. (1994) Fmr1 knockout mice: a model to study fragile X mental retardation. The Dutch-Belgian Fragile X consortium. Cell 78 (1):23–33
5. Castren M et al (2005) Altered differentiation of neural stem cells in fragile X syndrome. Proc Natl Acad Sci U S A 102(49):17834–17839
6. Eiges R et al (2007) Developmental study of fragile X syndrome using human embryonic stem cells derived from preimplantation genetically diagnosed embryos. Cell Stem Cell 1 (5):568–577
7. Takahashi K et al (2007) Induction of pluripotent stem cells from adult human fibroblasts by defined factors. Cell 131(5):861–872
8. Urbach A et al (2010) Differential modeling of fragile X syndrome by human embryonic stem

cells and induced pluripotent stem cells. Cell Stem Cell 6(5):407–411
9. Sheridan SD et al (2011) Epigenetic characterization of the FMR1 gene and aberrant neurodevelopment in human induced pluripotent stem cell models of fragile X syndrome. PLoS One 6(10):e26203
10. Lancaster MA et al (2013) Cerebral organoids model human brain development and microcephaly. Nature 501(7467):373–379
11. Braat S, Kooy RF (2014) Fragile X syndrome neurobiology translates into rational therapy. Drug Discov Today 19(4):510–519
12. Santos AR, Kanellopoulos AK, Bagni C (2014) Learning and behavioral deficits associated with the absence of the fragile X mental retardation protein: what a fly and mouse model can teach us. Learn Mem 21(10):543–555
13. Telias M, Ben-Yosef D (2014) Modeling neurodevelopmental disorders using human pluripotent stem cells. Stem Cell Rev 10 (4):494–511
14. Ascano M Jr et al (2012) FMRP targets distinct mRNA sequence elements to regulate protein expression. Nature 492(7429):382–386
15. Brennan TJ et al (1997) Sound-induced seizures in serotonin 5-HT2c receptor mutant mice. Nat Genet 16(4):387–390
16. Huber KM et al (2002) Altered synaptic plasticity in a mouse model of fragile X mental retardation. Proc Natl Acad Sci U S A 99 (11):7746–7750
17. Bear MF, Huber KM, Warren ST (2004) The mGluR theory of fragile X mental retardation. Trends Neurosci 27(7):370–377
18. Deng PY et al (2013) FMRP regulates neurotransmitter release and synaptic information transmission by modulating action potential duration via BK channels. Neuron 77 (4):696–711
19. Lohith TG et al (2013) Is metabotropic glutamate receptor 5 upregulated in prefrontal cortex in fragile X syndrome? Mol Autism 4(1):15
20. Telias M et al (2015) Functional deficiencies in fragile X neurons derived from human embryonic stem cells. J Neurosci 35 (46):15295–15306
21. Min WW et al (2009) Elevated glycogen synthase kinase-3 activity in Fragile X mice: key metabolic regulator with evidence for treatment potential. Neuropharmacology 56 (2):463–472
22. Guo W et al (2012) Inhibition of GSK3beta improves hippocampus-dependent learning and rescues neurogenesis in a mouse model of fragile X syndrome. Hum Mol Genet 21 (3):681–691
23. Telias M et al (2015) Molecular mechanisms regulating impaired neurogenesis of fragile X syndrome human embryonic stem cells. Stem Cells Dev 24(20):2353–2365
24. Braat S, Kooy RF (2015) Insights into GABAAergic system deficits in fragile X syndrome lead to clinical trials. Neuropharmacology 88:48–54
25. He Q et al (2014) The developmental switch in GABA polarity is delayed in fragile X mice. J Neurosci 34(2):446–450
26. D'Hulst C et al (2009) Expression of the GABAergic system in animal models for fragile X syndrome and fragile X associated tremor/ataxia syndrome (FXTAS). Brain Res 1253:176–183
27. Telias M, Segal M, Ben-Yosef D (2016) Immature responses to GABA in fragile X neurons derived from human embryonic stem cells. Front Cell Neurosci 10:121
28. Telias M, Ben-Yosef D (2015) Neural stem cell replacement: a possible therapy for neurodevelopmental disorders? Neural Regen Res 10 (2):180–182
29. Xie N et al (2016) Reactivation of FMR1 by CRISPR/Cas9-mediated deletion of the expanded CGG-repeat of the fragile X chromosome. PLoS One 11(10):e0165499
30. Park CY et al (2015) Reversion of FMR1 methylation and silencing by editing the triplet repeats in fragile X iPSC-derived neurons. Cell Rep 13(2):234–241
31. Liu XS et al (2018) Rescue of fragile X syndrome neurons by DNA methylation editing of the FMR1 gene. Cell 172(5):979–992 e6

Part II

FX Premutation

Chapter 14

Pathophysiology Mechanisms in Fragile-X Primary Ovarian Insufficiency

Shai E. Elizur, Moran Friedman Gohas, Olga Dratviman-Storobinsky, and Yoram Cohen

Abstract

Women who carry the FMR1 premutation may suffer from ongoing deterioration of ovarian function. The lucidity of the molecular mechanism of FXTAS is emerging and findings from research in the field of FXTAS could elucidate the pathogenesis of FXPOI. To date there are three possible mechanisms for ovarian dysfunction in FMR1 permutation carriers. The first is the RNA toxic gain-of-function mechanism initiating loss of function of over 30 specific RNA-binding proteins. The second is associated to the formation of an abnormal polyglycine-containing protein (FMRpolyG), and the third is related to novel lncRNAs, named FMR4 and FMR6. Herein we describe our laboratory methodology, focusing on the culturing and manipulation of granulosa cells from human female premutation carriers, trying to reveal the actual possible mechanisms liable to FXPOI. Detecting the precise pathways in premutation carrier might facilitate in offering these women the opportunity to make an informed decision regarding their reproductive and family planning.

Key words FXPOI, Granulosa cells, FMR1, FMR4, FMR6, FMRpolyG, RNA toxic gain-of-function, FMR1 premutation carriers

1 Introduction

An abnormal expansion of CGG trinucleotide repeats in the 5′-untranslated region of the *fragile X mental retardation 1 (FMR1)* gene located at Xq27.3 cause different genetic disorders according to the size of the repeat expansion [1, 2]. Patients with the full mutation (≥200 CGG-repeat) are accompanied by silencing of the *FMR1* promoter and absent of FMRP, which ultimately results in alterations of the brain synaptic plasticity [3, 4]. Expansion above the normal range (<55 repeats) toward the so-called premutation (PM) carrier state (55–199 repeats) is associated with increased risk for fragile X-associated primary ovarian insufficiency

Grant Sponsor: Azrieli research foundation Canada Israel

Dalit Ben-Yosef and Yoav Mayshar (eds.), *Fragile-X Syndrome: Methods and Protocols*, Methods in Molecular Biology, vol. 1942, https://doi.org/10.1007/978-1-4939-9080-1_14,

(FXPOI) in females [5, 6] and fragile X-associated tremor/ataxia syndrome (FXTAS) predominantly in males [7, 8]. The most immediate and significant consequence of FXPOI is reduced fertility [9, 10]. Consistently, females with PM alleles show normal or slightly reduced levels of FMRP and elevated FMR1 mRNA levels [3]. Expression of 88 CGG repeats in human granulosa cell (GC) line COV-434 was shown to cause cell damage/death to human GCs [11]. Similarly, increased expression of FMR1 mRNA in the ovary has been seen in all PM mouse models [12, 13]. In our recent study, FMR1 expression levels were measured in human GCs. There was a significant nonlinear association between the CGG repeats size, the FMR1 mRNA levels and the number of retrieved oocytes. The lowest number of retrieved oocytes and the highest level of mRNA were seen in women with mid-size CGG repeats (80–120). These results support the proposed RNA toxic gain-of-function mechanism [14]. To date, there are three possible mechanisms for Ovarian Dysfunction in PM Carriers. The first is the RNA gain-of-function hypothesis, which was first recognized in myotonic dystrophy type 1 and 2 [15]. In FXTAS and FXPOI, the expanded CGG repeats are predicted to sequester over 30 specific RNA-binding proteins directly or through a protein partner, many critical for normal cell function, such as lamin A/C, Pura, hnRNP, Sam68, and drosha [8, 12, 16]. Loss of function of these proteins in cells could compromise their normal functions, which would ultimately cause the symptoms and lead to early follicular loss. The second mechanism is related to the production of a polyglycine-containing protein [17] Todd et al. demonstrated that CGG repeats trigger repeat associated non-AUG initiated (RAN) translation of a cryptic polyglycine-containing protein, named FMRpolyG [18]. FMRpolyG accumulates in ubiquitin-positive inclusions in Drosophila, cell culture, mouse disease models, and FXTAS patient brains. Inclusions were also found in ovarian stromal cells of a PM women. Surprisingly, no inclusions were found in follicles [19]. Long noncoding (lnc) RNAs are the third possible mechanism that may involve the regulation of gene transcription/translation. Khalil et al. and Pastori et al. have reported the discovery of novel lncRNAs, named FMR4 and FMR6 that originate from the FMR1 gene locus [20–22]. FMR4 expression, similarly to FMR1, was found to be downregulated in brain tissue from FXS patients and upregulated in PM carriers. FMR4 and FMR6 were suggested to regulate FMR1 stability, splicing, subcellular localization, and translational efficiency in FXTAS [21]. Recently, we found that FMR6 is expressed in GCs from PM carriers and control. Both FMR1 mRNA and FMR6 lncRNA showed increased accumulation in GCs from PM carriers in the mid-range (80–120 CGG repeats) [23]. There are three common Knock In (KI) mouse models used to study FXTAS and FXPOI [12] as well as a Knock Out (KO) mouse and rat models representing the full mutation form. Within the KI models are CGGnih females containing a 130-repeat tract [24]. For repeat instability and the overexpression of FMRP study the YAC-TG296 (90-repeats) was found suitable [25]. The third KI model is the CGGdut, with an expanded 98-repeat. This model shows instability upon transmission and the biochemical, phenotypic, and neuropathological characteristics of FXTAS [26]. The rat model shows the potential of this model in understanding the toxic effect of the PM. Nonhuman primates (NHPs) offer a clinically relevant model system. One of the limitations in the NHPs model for FXPOI is that there are no known naturally occurring animal models with FMR1 repeat mutations. Thus, screening might be expensive and unlikely to yield sufficient animal numbers for meaningful studies. Producing Patient-specific induced pluripotent stem cells (iPSCs) derived from adult somatic cells and which have differentiated into GC-like cells with an elevated number of CGG repeats, might provide an option for generating an abundance of material for exploring FXPOI mechanisms. However, this research has not been extended to human iPSCs [27]. Human GCs can impart substantial information on human folliculogenesis and therefore are a compatible model for PM carriers. Moreover, human cell line transfected with expanded CGG repeats might offer an independent long-term model. Cross-referencing the findings between these two models might provide a nonlimited system for future studies.

2 Materials

2.1 Cell Culture

1. Dulbecco's modified Eagle's medium (DMEM) 1 g/l D-glucose (low glucose) with sodium pyruvate 110 mg/l.
2. Certified fetal bovine serum (FBS), heat inactivated.
3. Penicillin–streptomycin 10 mg/ml, stock solution.
4. L-glutamine 29.9 mg/ml in saline, stock solution.

2.2 qRT-PCR

1. SYBR Green FAST.
2. Primers:
   (a) h-FMR1_F: 5′-AACAAAGGACAGCATCGCTAATG-3′.
   (b) h-FMR1_R: 5′-CAAACGCAACTGGTCTACTTCCT-3′.
   (c) h-HPRT_F: 5′-AGATGGTCAAGGTCGCAAGCT-3′.
   (d) h-HPRT_R: 5′-TCAAATCCAACAAAGTCTGGCTTA-3′.
   (e) h-FMR4_F: 5′-ACC AAA CCA AAC CAA ACC AA-3′.
   (f) h-FMR4_R: 5′-GTG GGA AAT CAA ATG CAT CC-3′.
   (g) h-FMR6_F: 5′-AGC ACT TCA GGG CAG ATT TT-3′.
   (h) h-FMR6_R: 5′-TGG TGA ATG ATC ACC CAA TG-3′.

2.3 Immunostaining

1. Mounting medium containing the nuclear dye DAPI.

3 Methods

3.1 Mural GC Extraction and Purification

1. Place the 50 ml tube containing the follicular fluid collected from woman undergoing IVF treatments, for 10 min in room temperature (RT) in order to allow cells to settle by gravity.
2. Carefully remove the top medium, avoiding granulosa cells loss. Exclude any blood clots if detected and resuspend the cells in phosphate-buffered solution (1× PBS).
3. Allow the cells to settle by gravity for an additional 5 min.
4. Repeat **step 2** for 2–3 cycles, until the medium becomes clear.
5. The cells obtained are purified using Ficoll-Hypaque gradient, and then washed with PBS before centrifugation at 70 × *g* for 8 min.
6. Store the purified GCs of each patient at −80 °C until being assayed or proceed to cell culture [28].

3.2 Cumulus GC Extraction and Purification

1. After oocyte retrieval, place 200 μl of hyaluronidase (8 U/ 100 μl), gently pipet and once separated, remove the cumulus cells from the cumulus–oocyte complex.
2. Centrifuge at 200 × *g* for 5 min at RT [28].

3.3 Mural and Cumulus Granulosa Cell Culture

1. Prepare GCs culture medium: DMEM medium with 5% fetal bovine serum (FBS), 1% penicillin–streptomycin (2 mg/ 100 ml), and 1% of L-glutamine (6 mg/100 ml) (*see* Subheading 2.1 and **Note 1**).
2. Plate the preovulatory GCs that had been obtained from follicles during the IVF procedure into culture at a density of 100×10^3 cells/well of 6-well plates in culture medium (*see* **Notes 1–3** and Subheading 2.1).
3. After 4 days of medium exchange, replace the culture medium with fresh culture medium with 1 U/ml FSH (*see* **Note 3**).
4. After 2 days of medium with 1 U/ml FSH exchange, apply trypsin–EDTA 0.25% for 5 min followed by adding culture medium and collecting the suspended cells. Then centrifuge at 200 × *g* for 5 min and aspire the upper medium. Resuspend the pellet according to the analysis procedure planned and store at −80 °C (*see* **Notes 4** and **5**).

3.4 RNA Extraction from GCs

1. Extracted total RNA from GCs or WBCs by TRIzol reagent and a Mini RNA Isolation I Kit according to the manufacturer's instructions.

2. Convert total RNA to cDNA using a cDNA synthesis KIT according to the manufacturer's instructions: 42 °C for 30 min followed by 95 °C for 2 min with random hexamer primers in 20 μl total volume reaction. (For specific cDNA of lncRNA transcripts *see* **Note 6**).

3.5 Real-Time Quantitative PCR (RT-qPCR)

1. StepOne Software v2.2.2 is used for RT-qPCR.
2. Reaction is performed in a 10 μl volume, containing 1 μl cDNA (25 ng/μl final concentration), 0.5 μM each of the forward and reverse primers, and buffer is included in the Master Mix (*see* Subheading 2.2).
3. Cycling conditions include an initial denaturation step of 95 °C for 10 min followed by 50 cycles of 1 min at 95 °C and 1 min of annealing and extension at 60 °C.
4. Gene expression is normalized to housekeeping gene, human hypoxanthine guanine phosphoribosyltransferase and glyceraldehyde 3-phosphate dehydrogenase (GAPDH) as loading controls.
5. Threshold cycle efficiency corrections are calculated, and melting curves are obtained using cDNA for each individual-gene PCR assay; standard curves are obtained using untreated sample cDNA for each gene PCR assay.
6. The results are quantified by the comparative threshold cycle (Ct) method.$\Delta\Delta$Ct = ΔCt (sample) − ΔCt (reference gene) (DATA assist Software v2.2.2, Applied Biosystems).

3.6 Immunofluorescence

1. Grow cells on coverslips, wash with PBS and fix for 20 min in 4% PFA.
2. Permeabilize cells with 0.5% Triton X-100 for 15 min.
3. After blocking in 5% BSA for 60 min, immunostain cells for 1 h with a primary antibody at room temperture.
4. After subsequent washes with 1× PBS, incubate the cells for 1 h with secondary fluorescent antibody at room temperture.
5. Counterstain with DAPI—After PBS washes, coverslips should be carefully inverted to a drop of fluorescence mounting medium containing the nuclear dye DAPI (*see* Subheading 2.3) on a fluorescent microscope slides. The slides can be viewed immediately or stored in the dark at 4 °C for up to a month.

4 Notes

1. The culture medium should be warmed prior to use (37 °C).
2. Follicular fluid from woman undergoing IVF procedure usually provided an amount of cells sufficient to seed four wells.

3. Do not replace the culture medium with FSH for 48 h.
4. For RNA extraction storing the samples in 0.5 ml of TRIzol at −80 °C provided an impressive yield.
5. It is possible to store the cells in 0.5 ml of 1× PBS at −80 °C for protein analysis methods.
6. For specific cDNA of lncRNA transcripts of FMR gene (FMR4 and FMR6), instead of random primer specific primer of single strand should be used) [21].

References

1. Rousseau F, Heitz D, Biancalana V, Blumenfeld S, Kretz C, Boue J, Tommerup N, Van Der Hagen C, DeLozier-Blanchet C, Croquette MF et al (1991) Direct diagnosis by DNA analysis of the fragile X syndrome of mental retardation. N Engl J Med 325(24):1673–1681. https://doi.org/10.1056/NEJM199112123252401
2. Rovozzo R, Korza G, Baker MW, Li M, Bhattacharyya A, Barbarese E, Carson JH (2016) CGG repeats in the 5'UTR of FMR1 RNA regulate yranslation of other RNAs localized in the same RNA granules. PLoS One 11(12):e0168204. https://doi.org/10.1371/journal.pone.0168204
3. Willemsen R, Levenga J, Oostra BA (2011) CGG repeat in the FMR1 gene: size matters. Clin Genet 80(3):214–225. https://doi.org/10.1111/j.1399-0004.2011.01723.x
4. Saul RA, Tarleton JC (1993) In: Adam MP, Ardinger HH, Pagon RA et al (eds) FMR1-related disorders. GeneReviews((R)), Seattle, WA
5. Peprah E (2014) Understanding decreased fertility in women carriers of the FMR1 premutation: a possible mechanism for Fragile X-associated primary ovarian insufficiency (FXPOI). Reprod Health 11:67. https://doi.org/10.1186/1742-4755-11-67
6. Coffey SM, Cook K, Tartaglia N, Tassone F, Nguyen DV, Pan R, Bronsky HE, Yuhas J, Borodyanskaya M, Grigsby J, Doerflinger M, Hagerman PJ, Hagerman RJ (2008) Expanded clinical phenotype of women with the FMR1 premutation. Am J Med Genet A 146A(8):1009–1016. https://doi.org/10.1002/ajmg.a.32060
7. Hall DA, O'Keefe JA (2012) Fragile x-associated tremor ataxia syndrome: the expanding clinical picture, pathophysiology, epidemiology, and update on treatment. Tremor Other Hyperkinet Mov (N Y) 2:tre-02-56-352-1. https://doi.org/10.7916/D8HD7TDS
8. Kong HE, Zhao J, Xu S, Jin P, Jin Y (2017) Fragile X-associated tremor/ataxia syndrome: from molecular pathogenesis to development of therapeutics. Front Cell Neurosci 11:128. https://doi.org/10.3389/fncel.2017.00128
9. Allen EG, Sullivan AK, Marcus M, Small C, Dominguez C, Epstein MP, Charen K, He W, Taylor KC, Sherman SL (2007) Examination of reproductive aging milestones among women who carry the FMR1 premutation. Hum Reprod 22(8):2142–2152. https://doi.org/10.1093/humrep/dem148
10. Streuli I, Fraisse T, Ibecheole V, Moix I, Morris MA, de Ziegler D (2009) Intermediate and premutation FMR1 alleles in women with occult primary ovarian insufficiency. Fertil Steril 92(2):464–470. https://doi.org/10.1016/j.fertnstert.2008.07.007
11. Hubayter ZR, Tong ZB, Popat V, Hagerman PJ, Troendle J, Nelson LM (2009) Fragile X associated primary ovarian insufficiency (FXPOI): ovarian phenotype and <em>FMR1</em> RNA toxic gain of function in human granulosa cells. Fertil Steril 92(3):S6–S7. https://doi.org/10.1016/j.fertnstert.2009.07.025
12. Sherman SL, Curnow EC, Easley CA, Jin P, Hukema RK, Tejada MI, Willemsen R, Usdin K (2014) Use of model systems to understand the etiology of fragile X-associated primary ovarian insufficiency (FXPOI). J Neurodev Disord 6(1):26. https://doi.org/10.1186/1866-1955-6-26
13. Hoffman GE, Le WW, Entezam A, Otsuka N, Tong ZB, Nelson L, Flaws JA, McDonald JH, Jafar S, Usdin K (2012) Ovarian abnormalities in a mouse model of fragile X primary ovarian insufficiency. J Histochem Cytochem 60(6):439–456. https://doi.org/10.1369/0022155412441002

14. Elizur SE, Lebovitz O, Derech-Haim S, Dratviman-Storobinsky O, Feldman B, Dor J, Orvieto R, Cohen Y (2014) Elevated levels of FMR1 mRNA in granulosa cells are associated with low ovarian reserve in FMR1 premutation carriers. PLoS One 9(8):e105121. https://doi.org/10.1371/journal.pone.0105121
15. Fardaei M, Rogers MT, Thorpe HM, Larkin K, Hamshere MG, Harper PS, Brook JD (2002) Three proteins, MBNL, MBLL and MBXL, co-localize in vivo with nuclear foci of expanded-repeat transcripts in DM1 and DM2 cells. Hum Mol Genet 11(7):805–814
16. Sofola OA, Jin P, Qin Y, Duan R, Liu H, de Haro M, Nelson DL, Botas J (2007) RNA-binding proteins hnRNP A2/B1 and CUGBP1 suppress fragile X CGG premutation repeat-induced neurodegeneration in a Drosophila model of FXTAS. Neuron 55 (4):565–571. https://doi.org/10.1016/j.neuron.2007.07.021
17. Zu T, Gibbens B, Doty NS, Gomes-Pereira M, Huguet A, Stone MD, Margolis J, Peterson M, Markowski TW, Ingram MA, Nan Z, Forster C, Low WC, Schoser B, Somia NV, Clark HB, Schmechel S, Bitterman PB, Gourdon G, Swanson MS, Moseley M, Ranum LP (2011) Non-ATG-initiated translation directed by microsatellite expansions. Proc Natl Acad Sci U S A 108(1):260–265. https://doi.org/10.1073/pnas.1013343108
18. Todd PK, Oh SY, Krans A, He F, Sellier C, Frazer M, Renoux AJ, Chen KC, Scaglione KM, Basrur V, Elenitoba-Johnson K, Vonsattel JP, Louis ED, Sutton MA, Taylor JP, Mills RE, Charlet-Berguerand N, Paulson HL (2013) CGG repeat-associated translation mediates neurodegeneration in fragile X tremor ataxia syndrome. Neuron 78(3):440–455. https://doi.org/10.1016/j.neuron.2013.03.026
19. Buijsen RA, Visser JA, Kramer P, Severijnen EA, Gearing M, Charlet-Berguerand N, Sherman SL, Berman RF, Willemsen R, Hukema RK (2016) Presence of inclusions positive for polyglycine containing protein, FMRpolyG, indicates that repeat-associated non-AUG translation plays a role in fragile X-associated primary ovarian insufficiency. Hum Reprod 31 (1):158–168. https://doi.org/10.1093/humrep/dev280
20. Khalil AM, Faghihi MA, Modarresi F, Brothers SP, Wahlestedt C (2008) A novel RNA transcript with antiapoptotic function is silenced in fragile X syndrome. PLoS One 3(1):e1486. https://doi.org/10.1371/journal.pone.0001486
21. Pastori C, Peschansky VJ, Barbouth D, Mehta A, Silva JP, Wahlestedt C (2014) Comprehensive analysis of the transcriptional landscape of the human FMR1 gene reveals two new long noncoding RNAs differentially expressed in Fragile X syndrome and Fragile X-associated tremor/ataxia syndrome. Hum Genet 133(1):59–67. https://doi.org/10.1007/s00439-013-1356-6
22. Pastori C, Wahlestedt C (2012) Involvement of long noncoding RNAs in diseases affecting the central nervous system. RNA Biol 9 (6):860–870. https://doi.org/10.4161/rna.20482
23. Elizur SE, Dratviman-Storobinsky O, Derech-Haim S, Lebovitz O, Dor J, Orvieto R, Cohen Y (2016) FMR6 may play a role in the pathogenesis of fragile X-associated premature ovarian insufficiency. Gynecol Endocrinol 32 (4):334–337. https://doi.org/10.3109/09513590.2015.1116508
24. Entezam A, Biacsi R, Orrison B, Saha T, Hoffman GE, Grabczyk E, Nussbaum RL, Usdin K (2007) Regional FMRP deficits and large repeat expansions into the full mutation range in a new Fragile X premutation mouse model. Gene 395(1–2):125–134. https://doi.org/10.1016/j.gene.2007.02.026
25. Lu C, Lin L, Tan H, Wu H, Sherman SL, Gao F, Jin P, Chen D (2012) Fragile X premutation RNA is sufficient to cause primary ovarian insufficiency in mice. Hum Mol Genet 21 (23):5039–5047. https://doi.org/10.1093/hmg/dds348
26. Bontekoe CJ, Bakker CE, Nieuwenhuizen IM, van der Linde H, Lans H, de Lange D, Hirst MC, Oostra BA (2001) Instability of a (CGG) 98 repeat in the Fmr1 promoter. Hum Mol Genet 10(16):1693–1699
27. Kang Y, Cheng MJ, Xu CJ (2011) Secretion of oestrogen from murine-induced pluripotent stem cells co-cultured with ovarian granulosa cells in vitro. Cell Biol Int 35(9):871–874. https://doi.org/10.1042/CBI20100737
28. Maman E, Yung Y, Cohen B, Konopnicki S, Dal Canto M, Fadini R, Kanety H, Kedem A, Dor J, Hourvitz A (2011) Expression and regulation of sFRP family members in human granulosa cells. Mol Hum Reprod 17 (7):399–404. https://doi.org/10.1093/molehr/gar010

Chapter 15

Fragile X-Associated Tremor/Ataxia Syndrome (FXTAS)

Marwa Zafarullah and Flora Tassone

Abstract

Individuals carrying an *FMR1* expansion between 55 and 200 CGG repeats, are at risk of developing the Fragile X-associated tremor/ataxia syndrome (FXTAS), a late onset neurodegenerative disorder characterized by cerebellar gait ataxia, intentional tremor, neuropathy, parkinsonism, cognitive decline, and psychological disorders, such as anxiety and depression. In addition, brain atrophy, white matter disease, and hyperintensities of the middle cerebellar peduncles can also be present. The neuropathological distinct feature of FXTAS is represented by the presence of eosinophilic intranuclear inclusions in neurons and astrocytes throughout the brain and in other tissues. In this chapter, protocols for available diagnostic tools, in both humans and mice, the clinical features and the basic molecular mechanisms leading to FXTAS and the animal models proposed to study this disorder are discussed.

Key words Tremor, Ataxia, FXTAS, *FMR1*, FMRP, qRT-PCR, TP-PCR

1 Introduction

The human *FMR1* gene spans approximately 38 kb of genomic DNA, consisting of 17 exons [1] and it undergoes alternative splicing involving multiple exons [2]. The length of the trinucleotide CGG repeats in the promoter defines different allele categories [3]. Those harboring between 55 and 200 CGG repeats, are named premutations which are unstable upon transmission and have the propensity to expand into a full mutation allele in following generations [4, 5]. Premutation alleles have a prevalence among the general population of ~1 in 110–260 females and ~1 in 400–850 males; however, the prevalence can vary depending on ethnicity [6], being the highest in Colombia and Israel [7, 8].

Many studies in recent years have reported that premutation carriers are at increased risk for a number of medical problems, which include, but are not limited, to hypertension [9], central pain sensitivity syndrome, sleep problems, restless legs syndrome (RLS) [10], migraine [11], and gait issues [12]. In addition, the presence of a premutation can also cause developmental problems

Dalit Ben-Yosef and Yoav Mayshar (eds.), *Fragile-X Syndrome: Methods and Protocols*, Methods in Molecular Biology, vol. 1942, https://doi.org/10.1007/978-1-4939-9080-1_15,

such as ASD and ADHD particularly in young boys [13–15], cognitive [16] and psychiatric features, including anxiety [17, 18] and depression [19] in both children and adults.

Carriers of a premutation allele are at the risk of developing both Fragile X-associated tremor/ataxia syndrome (FXTAS) and Fragile X-associated primary ovarian insufficiency (FXPOI). About 40% of male carriers over the age of 50 develop FXTAS. The penetrance is age related, such that 75% of men ≥80 years of age are affected [20]. Approximately 8% of female carriers develop FXTAS [21]. In addition, approximately 20% of female carriers of a premutation allele develop Fragile X-associated primary ovarian insufficiency, a loss of normal ovary function before the age of 40, compared to 1% women in the general population [22, 23].

The main clinical features of fragile X-associated tremor/ataxia syndrome (FXTAS) include the presence of gait ataxia and intentional tremor [24]. Observed imaging abnormalities comprise global brain atrophy and cerebellar white matter changes, including hyperintensity of the middle cerebellar peduncles (MCP) [25, 26].

Male premutation carriers over age 50, with and without FXTAS, have increased rates of anxiety, hostility, apathy, irritability, agitation, obsessive compulsiveness, and depression [27], while female carriers, with and without FXTAS, show a high rate of depressive symptoms as compared to normal individuals [28]. Importantly, female premutation carriers, particularly those with core features of FXTAS, present with thyroid dysfunction (17% in the non-FXTAS group and 50% in the FXTAS group) [29].

Individuals with a premutation allele have up to eightfold elevation of *FMR1* mRNA expression levels, which positively correlate with the (CGG)n repeat length. Interestingly, although *FMR1* transcript levels increase with increased CGG repeats, the levels of FMRP gradually decreases with increasing (CGG)n length due to decreased translational efficiency of long expanded CGG alleles [30, 31]. Thus, differently from fragile X syndrome (FXS), which is caused by the lack of FMRP, FXTAS and the premutation disorders arise through a distinct and different molecular mechanism involving the presence of elevated levels of *FMR1* expanded CGG-repeat transcripts, leading to RNA toxicity.

Various models have been proposed to explain the disease mechanisms for FXTAS. The first proposed model was the RNA gain-of-function or sequestration model based on the proposed myotonic dystrophy model [32]. This model postulates that the excessive expanded CGG containing mRNA binds a number of CGG binding proteins which sequestration affects their normal cellular functions [24]. Among these proteins, Sam68 is an RNA-binding protein involved in alternative splicing regulation that colocalize with CGG aggregates [33] and DGCR8 which with Drosha forms a protein complex involved in the biogenesis of miRNA. As result reduced levels of many miRNAs but increased levels of their precursors have been detected in brain tissues derived from individuals with FXTAS [34].

Repeat-associated non-AUG (RAN) translation, is an alternative proposed mechanism for explaining the pathogenesis of FXTAS [35], which posits that the translation of the *FMR1* mRNA occurs upstream of the expanded repeat generating three different homopolypeptides. However, among the three, the polyarginine (FMRpolyG) is produced more efficiently and results in a toxic homopolypeptide that can affect cellular functions and consequently plays a role in FXTAS [36, 37].

The third proposed mechanism is based on DNA damage response model leading to the formation of secondary R-loop structures. The transcription of highly GC-rich region, such as the 5′ UTR region of *FMR1* gene, promotes the formation of R-loops in which the nascent RNA forms a stable RNA–DNA hybrid with the template DNA strand. A recent study shows that R-loops formed over CGG repeats at endogenous *FMR1* locus may be susceptible to structural complexities, including hairpin formation, that is not commonly associated with other R-loops. Moreover the R-loop formation increases with higher expression levels of *FMR1* gene. [38].

The abovementioned models are not mutually exclusive and likely they all contribute to the development of FXTAS, but how exactly they lead and what is their relative contribution to the pathogenesis of this disorder remain unknown.

1.1 Clinical Features and Methods for the Diagnosis of FXTAS

For the diagnostic criteria of FXTAS (Table 1), tremor and ataxia are considered the main clinical features for a definite diagnosis of FXTAS. At the molecular level the presence of an expanded allele from the gray through the premutation range is required for the diagnosis of FXTAS [39].

Three categories, termed as "definite," "probable," and "possible," are used in the diagnosis of FXTAS. "Definite" indicates the presence of one major radiological sign plus one major clinical symptom. "Probable" indicates the presence of either one major radiology sign plus one minor clinical symptom or two major clinical symptoms. "Possible" indicates the presence of one minor radiology sign plus one major clinical symptom (Table 1). In addition, the diagnosis of FXTAS can also be clarified by the stage of disease, which provides information of the impact of disease on activities of daily living. Six FXTAS stages have been described and they include stage 0: normal function; stage 1: subtle or questionable signs such as subtle tremor or mild balance problems, with no interference in ADLs; stage 2: minor but clear tremor and/or balance problems with minor interference with ADLs; stage 3: moderate tremor and/or balance problems and occasional falls with significant interference in ADLs; stage 4: severe tremor and /or balance problems (uses cane or walker); and stage 6: bedridden.

Table 1
Diagnostic Criteria of FXTAS

Diagnostic criteria		
Definite	Probable	Possible
One clinical major + [one radiological or pathological major]	Two clinical major or [one clinical minor + one radiological major]	One clinical major + one clinical or radiological minor
Molecular		
Required	*FMR1* mutation including the gray zone	
Clinical		
Major	Intention tremor, Cerebellar gait ataxia	
Minor	Parkinsonism, Neuropathy, Executive function deficit, >Moderate short term memory deficit.	
Neuropathology		
Major	Ubiquitin-positive intranuclear inclusions	
Radiological		
Major	MRI white matter lesions in MCPs or brainstem	
Minor	MRI cerebral white matter lesions, MRI white matter lesions in the splenium of the corpus callosum. >Moderate generalized brain atrophy	

1.2 Molecular Features and Methods for the Diagnosis of FXTAS

The molecular diagnosis of the FXTAS is based on the CGG repeat allele size length and specifically on the presence of premutation allele. Recently, the CGG range has been extended throughout the intermediate allele range [40] as it has been shown that the individuals carrying the gray zone expansion can be affected by FXTAS [41, 42]. Although the molecular diagnosis of fragile X syndrome and associated disorders is accomplished by the combination of polymerase chain reaction (PCR) and Southern blot analyses (Fig. 1), the size of the CGG repeat length and the molecular diagnosis of FXTAS are generally carried out by the PCR approach which can reliably estimate their exact CGG repeat number from the normal to the premutation range.

The conventional flanking or repeat-spanning PCR techniques use two locus-specific primers to amplify across the *FMR1* CGG repeats; however, these approaches do not allow for amplification of large premutation alleles and they do not provide information on the presence and distribution of the AGG interruptions. These old PCR methods that used slab-gel electrophoresis for the detection of the CGG-containing amplicons have been replaced by the more robust fluorescent PCRs and by capillary electrophoresis, for better allelic resolution and for a more accurate CGG-repeat sizing.

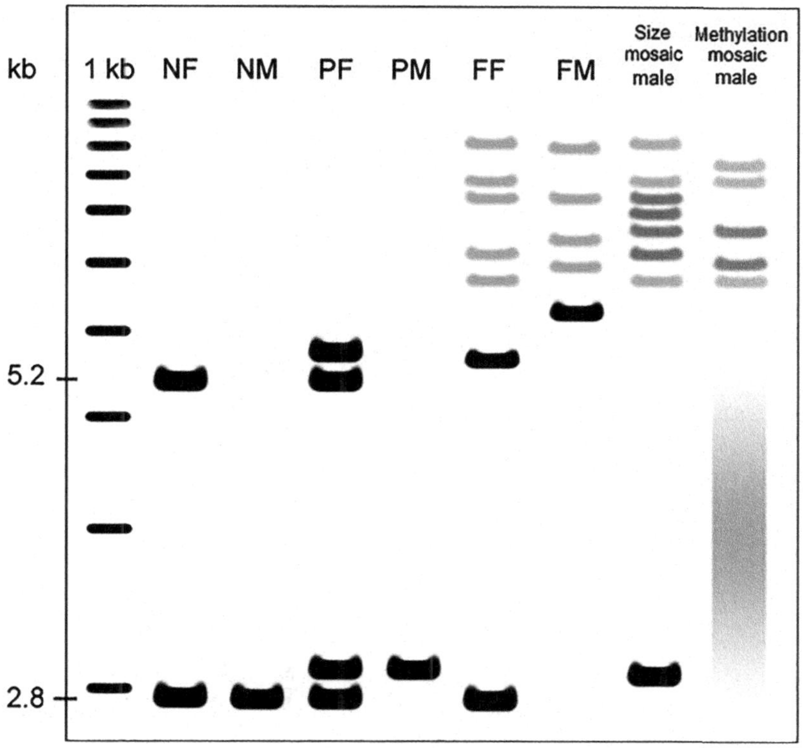

NF = Normal female
NM = Normal male
PF = Premutation female
PM = Premutation male
FF = Full mutation female
FM = Full mutation male

Fig. 1 Diagram of Southern blot analysis of genomic DNA showing different CGG band patterns of alleles throughout the CGG range (normal to full mutation) in both males and females. The DNA marker, 1 kb ladder, is shown in Lane 1. Normal unmethylated band (2.8 kb) and normal methylated band (5.2 kb) in a normal female are shown in lane 2. Normal male, and premutation female and male are shown in lane 3, 4, and 5, respectively. Lane 6 and 7 show a typical band pattern for full mutation female and full mutation male. In the last two lanes, 8 and 9, the mutation pattern of mosaic males, size, and methylation are depicted.

Indeed, a number of different PCR-based methods have been proposed over the years to overcome the failure of the amplification of large *FMR1* alleles due to their high CG content and to the tendency to form undenaturable secondary structures.

One important issue in common to all of the earlier assays is that they are not always able to resolve the apparent homozygosity in females, meaning that they cannot distinguish between the presence of two identical *FMR1* alleles within the normal range versus one normal allele and one, unamplified, full mutation allele. This obstacle was overcome by the use of the CGG/CCG primer [43] and by the development of a newer and more robust PCR-based approach, the triplet-primed PCR (TP-PCR) assay [44], which

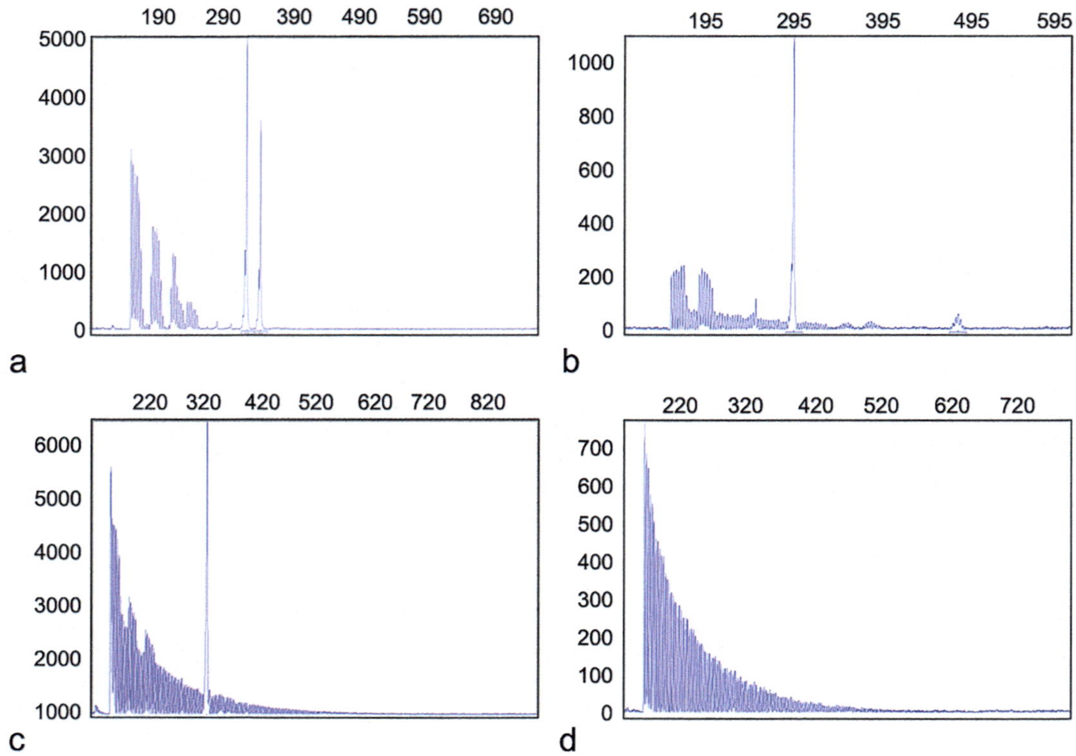

Fig. 2 Representative CE profiles of normal female (**a**), premutation female (**b**), full-mutation female (**c**), and full mutation male (**d**) using the CGG repeat primed PCR which generates, in addition to the full-length specific *FMR1* allele also many CGG repeat primed products, which are resolved by CE as a series of peaks on each electropherogram

currently represents an ideal tool for amplifying trinucleotide repeat expansions throughout the CGG repeat range in both males and females.

The triplet-primed PCR (TP-PCR) assay employs, in addition to two *FMR1*-specific primers, annealing outside the CGG repeat, the use of a CGG primer, which randomly anneals within the CGG repeat element. PCR amplification gives arise to a series of amplicons that are then visualized as a smear on an agarose gel [43] or as a series of peaks on capillary electrophoresis (CE) [44] [Fig. 2]. Several studies [44–47] have demonstrated that the TP-PCR provides results that are comparable to those obtained by the combined PCR-Southern blot approach, making it the method of choice for the diagnosis of FXS and Fragile X associated disorders, including FXTAS, in many laboratories worldwide. The TP-PCR also allows for the mapping of AGG interruptions, which enables to predict the risks of CGG expansion to a full mutation during mother-to-child transmission [5, 48], which is important for genetic counseling of women premutation carriers, further enhancing the reproductive decision-making process.

2 Materials

2.1 DNA Isolation from Human Blood, Cultured Cells and Tissues

1. RNase A.
2. Isopropanol.
3. 70% ethanol (*see* **Note 1**).
4. RBC Lysis Solution: 0.16 M ammonium chloride in 0.01 M Tris–HCl buffer, pH 7.2 (*see* **Note 2**).
5. Cell Lysis Solution: 10 mM Tris–HCl buffer, 1 mM EDTA, and 0.5% SDS (*see* **Note 3**).
6. DNA Hydration Solution: 1 mM EDTA, 10 mM Tris–HCI pH 7.5 (*see* **Note 4**).
7. Protein Precipitation Solution: 7.5 M ammonium acetate (*see* **Note 5**).

2.2 Triplet-Primed PCR (TP-PCR) in Human

1. GC-Rich AMP Buffer: 7.5 mM $MgCl_2$ and 7% w/w DMSO (*see* **Note 6**).
2. GC-Rich Polymerase Mix: 20 mM Tris–HCl pH 8.0, 100 mM KCl, 0.1 mM EDTA, 1 mM DTT, 0.5% Tween 20 (v/v), 0.5% Nonidet, P40 (v/v), and 50% glycerol (v/v) (*see* **Note 7**).
3. *FMR1* Forward, Reverse FAM-Primer.
4. *FMR1* CGG repeat-specific primer $(CGG)_5$.
5. Genomic DNA (positive control or nuclease-free H_2O for negative control).
6. Nuclease-free H_2O.
7. ROX 1000 Size Ladder.

2.3 Isolation of DNA from Mouse Tails

1. Tail Buffer: 50 mM Tris pH = 7.5, 10 mM EDTA, 150 mM NaCl, 1% SDS (*see* **Note 8**).
2. Proteinase K (10 mg/ml) (*see* **Note 9**).
3. 6 M NaCl (*see* **Note 10**).
4. Ethanol (100%, 70%).
5. Nuclease-free water.

2.4 CGG Repeat Sizing in Mouse

1. 5× Expand HF plus buffer with Mg: 25 mM TAPS [tris(hydroxymethyl)methylamino]propanesulfonic acid—HCl (pH 9.3 at 25 °C), 50 mM KCl, 2 mM $MgCl_2$, 1 mM β-mercaptoethanol, 200 μM dNTPs including [^{3}H]-dTTP and 15 nM primed M13 DNA.
2. 5 M betaine (*see* **Note 11**).
3. DMSO. Store at room temperature in the dark.
4. dNTP solution: 25 mM (*see* **Note 12**).
5. Primers: (*see* **Note 13**).

(a) Forward (5′-CGGAGGCGCCGCTGCCAGG-3′).
(b) Reverse (5′-TGCGGGCGCTCGAGGCCCAG-3′).

6. Expand High Fidelity plus PCR system Enzyme.
7. Nuclease-free water.

2.5 Quantitative Reverse Transcriptase PCR (qRT-PCR) of FMR1 mRNA

1. 10× PCR Buffer: 500 mM Tris–HCl pH 9.0, 15 mM $MgCl_2$, 220 mM $(NH_4)_2SO_4$, 2% triton x-100 (*see* **Note 14**).
2. 25 mM $MgCl_2$ (*see* **Note 15**).
3. dNTP (25 mM).
4. Hexamers (100 μM).
5. RNase Inhibitor (40 U/μl).
6. Mulv RT (200 U/μl).
7. DEPC H_2O.
8. *FMR1*-specific primers (100 μM).
9. Probe designed for a specific targeted region.
10. Taqman Master Mix.
11. 384-Well plate.
12. 96-Well plate.
13. Optical adhesive seal.

3 Methods

DNA isolation can be performed using standard reagents available from different companies like Qiagen Valencia.

3.1 DNA Isolation from Human Blood

1. Add 900 μl of RBC Lysis Solution into a 1.5 ml microcentrifuge tube and add 300 μl, whole blood mix by inverting ten times.
2. Incubate for 1 min at room temperature (15–25 °C) and invert at least once during the incubation.
3. Centrifuge for 20 s at 13,000–16,000 × *g* to pellet the white blood cells and remove the supernatant.
4. Vortex the tube vigorously to suspend the pellet in the residual liquid and then add 300 μl, Cell Lysis Solution, and pipet up and down to lyse the cells or vortex vigorously for 10 s.
5. To remove RNA, add 1.5 μl RNase A Solution and mix by inverting 25 times. Incubate for 15 min at 37 °C. Then incubate for 1 min on ice to quickly cool the sample.
6. Add 100 μl, Protein Precipitation Solution, and vortex vigorously for 20 s at high speed. Centrifuge for 1 min at 13,000–16,000 × *g*.

7. Pipet 300 μl isopropanol into a clean 1.5 ml tube and add the supernatant from the previous step by pouring carefully.
8. Mix by inverting gently 50 times until the DNA is visible as threads or a clump.
9. Centrifuge for 1 min at 13,000–16,000 × *g* and the DNA may be visible as a small white pellet.
10. Carefully discard the supernatant, and drain the tube by inverting on a clean piece of absorbent paper, taking care that the pellet remains in the tube.
11. Add 300 μl of 70% ethanol and invert several times to wash the DNA pellet.
12. Centrifuge for 1 min at 13,000–16,000 × *g*, remove the ethanol, and air-dry the pellet for 5 min.
13. Carefully discard the supernatant. Drain the tube. Add 100 μl DNA Hydration Solution and vortex for 5 s at medium speed to mix.
14. Incubate at 65 °C for 5 min to dissolve the DNA then incubate at room temperature overnight with gentle shaking. Samples can then be centrifuged briefly and transferred to a storage tube.

3.2 DNA Isolation from Cultured Cells

1. Harvest cells and determine the number of cells.
2. Take 1–2 × 10^6 cells in growth culture medium to a 1.5 ml microcentrifuge tube and centrifuge for 5 s at 13,000–16,000 × *g* to pellet cells.
3. Carefully discard the supernatant by pipetting or pouring, leaving approximately 20 μl residual liquid.
4. Now Vortex the tube vigorously to resuspend the cells in the residual supernatant and add 300 μl Cell Lysis Solution to the resuspended cells and pipet up and down or vortex on high speed for 10 s to lyse the cells.
5. To remove RNA, add 1.5 μl of RNase A Solution and mix by inverting 25 times. Incubate for 5 min at 37 °C. Incubate for 1 min on ice to quickly cool the sample.
6. Add 100 μl Protein Precipitation Solution and vortex vigorously for 20 s at high speed.
7. Pipet 300 μl isopropanol into a clean 1.5 ml microcentrifuge tube and add the supernatant from the previous step by pouring carefully.
8. Mix by inverting gently 50 times.
9. Centrifuge for 1 min at 13,000–16,000 × *g* and carefully discard the supernatant.

10. Drain the tube by inverting on a clean piece of absorbent paper, taking care that the pellet remains in the tube.
11. Add 300 μl of 70% ethanol and invert several times to wash the DNA pellet. Centrifuge for 1 min at 13,000–16,000 × *g*.
12. Carefully discard the supernatant and drain the tube on a clean piece of absorbent paper. Allow to air-dry for 5 min.
13. Add 100 μl of DNA Hydration Solution and vortex for 5 s at medium speed to mix.
14. Incubate at 65 °C for 1 h to dissolve the DNA. Samples can then be centrifuged briefly and transferred to a storage tube.

3.3 DNA Isolation from Tissue

1. Dissect tissue sample quickly and freeze in liquid nitrogen. Grind 5–10 mg or frozen or fresh tissue in liquid nitrogen with a mortar and pestle.
2. Add 300 μl Cell Lysis Solution into a 1.5 ml grinder tube on ice and add the ground tissue from the previous step.
3. Add 1.5 μl Proteinase K, mix by inverting 25 times, and incubate at 55 °C for 3 h or until tissue has completely lysed.
4. Add 1.5 μl RNase A Solution, and mix the sample by inverting 25 times. Incubate at 37 °C for 15–60 min and then cool down on ice quickly.
5. Add 100 μl Protein Precipitation Solution, and vortex vigorously for 20 s at high speed.
6. Centrifuge for 3 min at 13,000–16,000 × *g*.
7. Pipet 300 μl isopropanol into a clean 1.5 ml microcentrifuge tube and add the supernatant from the previous step by pouring carefully.
8. Mix by inverting gently 50 times and centrifuge for 1 min at 13,000–16,000 × *g*.
9. Carefully discard the supernatant and drain the tube by inverting on a clean piece of absorbent paper.
10. Add 300 μl of 70% ethanol and invert several times to wash the DNA pellet. Centrifuge for 1 min at 13,000–16,000 × *g*.
11. Carefully discard the supernatant. Drain the tube on a clean piece of absorbent paper, taking care that the pellet remains in the tube. Allow to air-dry for 5 min.
12. Add 100 μl DNA Hydration Solution and vortex for 5 s at medium speed to mix.
13. Incubate at room temperature (15–25 °C) overnight with gentle shaking. Ensure tube cap is tightly closed to avoid leakage. Samples can then be centrifuged briefly and transferred to a storage tube.

3.4 Triplet-Primed PCR (TP-PCR) in Human

1. The following volumes of the PCR mix are for one PCR-reaction: 11.45 µl of GC-rich AMP buffer, 0.5 µl of each primer: *FMR1* forward and *FMR1* reverse, 0.5 µl of *FMR1* CGG primer, 0.5 µl of nuclease-free H_2O, 0.05 µl of GC-rich polymerase mix, 2 µl of DNA sample. Total volume is 15 µl.
2. Initiate the PCR program and wait until the block has reached at least 103 °C before putting the tubes into the cycler machine. PCR conditions are as: 95 °C 5 min, 10 cycles (97 °C 35 s, 62 °C 35 s, 68 °C 4 min), 20 cycles (97 °C 35 s, 62 °C 35 s, 68 °C 4 min + 20 s/cycle), 72 °C 10 min, then hold at 4 °C or store at −20 °C.
3. The products can be analyzed on an agarose gel or by capillary electrophoresis using the Hi-Di/ROX-MW Ladder (Hi-Di/ROX solution).

3.5 Premutation Animal Models

Premutation mouse models, CGG knockin (CGG KI), were developed even before the discovery of the FXTAS, as they were designed to study the CGG repeat instability. These mouse models which express a CGG repeats in premutation range (81 CGG and 97 CGG), showed to stably inherited through generations compared to humans [49, 50]. However, later on, the same authors demonstrated CGG repeat instability upon both maternal and paternal transmission in the same KI mouse model [51]. Further, several transgenic mouse lines showed the length-dependent instability in the form of small expansions and contractions in both male and female transmissions over five generations [52].

Increased *FMR1* mRNA levels and intranuclear inclusions throughout the brain were observed in these mice [53]. A different knockin mouse model harboring an allele of 118 CGG repeats shows repeat instability and high expression levels of *FMR1 mRNA* and low level of FMRP. The large expansion into the full mutation in one single generation was observed in these mice [54]. However, no methylation of the promoter region has been detected thus far in any these mice [53–57]. CGG mice display heightened anxiety, deficits in motor coordination and impaired gait and represent the first FXTAS model that exhibits an ataxia phenotype as observed in patients [35, 56, 58–60].

A Drosophila model was generated by expressing 90 CGG repeats, which results in neuronal death of the peripheral and central nervous system [61]. Overexpression of Pur α, an RNA-binding protein expressed in the neuronal cytoplasm associates with (CGG)n RNA and suppress the eye neurodegeneration phenotype. This protein is present in the inclusions in Drosophila [62], as well as in human FXTAS brain [63] supporting the sequestration model of FXTAS as one of the mechanism leading to altered cellular function and ultimately neuronal cell death [62].

3.5.1 Isolation of DNA from Mouse Tails

1. Incubate tail in 300 μl tail buffer and 20 μl of Protease K (10 mg/ml) at 55 °C for 24 h.
2. Add 100 μl 6 M NaCl to the tail–buffer mixture and shake vigorously.
3. Spin at maximum speed for 10 min, collect the supernatant, and add 1 ml of 100% ethanol.
4. Mix it well and take out the DNA cloud formed with pipette and transfer into the tube containing 500 μl ethanol.
5. Spin at maximum speed for 7 min, discard supernatant, and dry the pellet.
6. Suspend the DNA pellet into nuclease-free water and store at −20 °C for further use.

3.5.2 CGG Repeat Sizing in Mouse

1. The following volumes for the PCR master mix are for one PCR-reaction: 10.5 μl of commercial water, 1 μl of 100 μM forward primer, 1 μl of 100 μM reverse primer, 0.5 μl of 25 mM dNTP mix, 1 μl of DMSO, 25 μl of 5 M betaine, 1 μl of Expand High Fidelity plus PCR system Enzyme, and 10 μl of 5× Expand HF plus buffer with Mg and 1 μl of DNA sample. The final volume is 50 μl.
2. Initiate the PCR program and wait until the block has reached at least 103 °C before putting the tubes into the cycler machine. PCR conditions are as follows: 95 °C 10 min, 35 cycles (95 °C 1 min, 65 °C 1 min, 75 °C 5 min), 75 °C 10 min, then hold at 10 °C or store at −20 °C until ready to analyze.
3. The products can be analyzed by 1.5% agarose gel electrophoresis. An approximate repeat length is calculated based on making a (logarithmic) standard curve.
4. For more accurate size determinations, the samples can be analyzed on a 6% polyacrylamide gel. Alternatively, if one the primer is FAM labeled, CGG sizing can be obtained on a capillary electrophoresis.

3.6 Analysis of mRNA Expression of Premutation Career by qRT-PCR

The premutation clinical involvements, including FXTAS are thought to be associated with increased level of CGG expanded *FMR1* mRNA. The level of increased mRNA can be quantified by quantitative reverse transcriptase PCR (qRT-PCR) [64].

3.6.1 Reverse Transcriptase: First Strand cDNA Synthesis

For making cDNA, PCR master mix should be made on ice to give sufficient volume for several RT-PCR reactions. The following volumes are for one PCR-reaction: 10 μl of 10× PCR buffer, 22 μl $MgCl_2$ at 25 mM, 4 μl of dNTP at 25 mM, 5 μl of hexamers at 100 μM, 1 μl of RNase Inhibitor at (40 U/μl), 1.25 μl of Mulv RT at 200 U/μl, and 51.75 μl of DEPC water.

1. No RT-PCR control reaction is as follows: 10 μl of 10× PCR buffer, 22 μl $MgCl_2$ at 25 mM, 4 μl of dNTP at 25 mM, 5 μl of hexamers at 100 μM, 1 μl of RNase Inhibitor at (40 U/μl, No Mulv) and 53 μl of DEPC water.
2. Five hundred nanograms of total RNA should be used for each RT reaction. To control for RT efficiency three total RNA concentrations should be used (i.e., 500 ng, 250 ng, 125 ng).
3. Initiate the PCR program and wait until the block has reached at least 103 °C before putting the tubes into the cycler machine. PCR conditions are as follow: 25 °C 10 min, 48 °C 40 min, 95 °C 5 min, then hold at 4 °C or store at −20 °C until ready to use.

3.6.2 Quantitative PCR (qPCR) of FMR1 mRNA

1. To analyze gene expression levels relate to a reference gene using the comparative method [64] prepare a primer–probe mixture (P/P) as follows: 152 μl DEPC H_2O, 8 μl probe (*FMR1* or reference gene) (100 μM), 40 μl Forward primer (100 μM), and 40 μl Reverse primer (100 μM). The final volume is 240 μl.
2. Prepare 7 μl of master mix which contains 6 μl of Taqman master mix plus 0.42 μl of H_2O and 0.58 μl of P/P. Add 5 μl of cDNA to each tube. The final volume is 12 μl. If you are using 96 or 384 plates, seal with foil.
3. Spin tunes or plates for 1 min at 2000 rpm or 860 × *g* at 4 °C.
4. Run the reaction in a 7300/7500 real-time PCR system.
5. Expression data can be analyzed as detailed in [64] or https://assets.thermofisher.com/TFS-Assets/LSG/manuals/cms_053412.pdf.

4 Notes

1. For 100 ml of 70% ethanol dissolve the 70 ml of 100% ethanol in 30 ml of water. For the higher volume the amount can be adjusted accordingly.
2. For 500 ml of RBC lysis buffer dissolve 4.15 g of ammonium chloride (53.491 g/mol) and 605 mg of Tris–HCl (121.14 g/mol) in a 450 ml of distilled water. Adjust the pH to 7.2 with HCl and bring the volume to 500 ml.
3. Dissolve 605 mg of Tris–HCl (121.14 g/mol), 146.12 mg of EDTA (292.24 g/mol), and 250 mg of SDS (288.372 g/mol) in 450 ml of water. After dissolving properly add up more distilled water and bring the volume to 500 ml.
4. Dissolve 146.12 mg of EDTA (292.24 g/mol) and 605 mg of Tris–HCl (121.14 g/mol) in 450 ml of water. Adjust the pH to 7.5 with HCl and bring the volume to 500 ml.

5. Dissolve 289 g of ammonium acetate (77.0825 g/mol) in 450 ml of water. After proper dissolving add the distilled water to bring the volume to 500 ml.
6. Dissolve 0.578 mg of $MgCl_2$ (77.0825 g/mol) and 70 mg of DMSO (78.13 g/mol) in 0.5 ml of water. After proper dissolving add the distilled water to make up the volume to 1 ml.
7. Add 200 μl of 1 M Tris–HCl pH 8.0, 74 mg of 1 M KCl, 100 μl of 10 mM EDTA, 10 μl of 1 mM DTT, 50 μl of Tween 20, 50 μl of Nonidet P40, and 500 μl of glycerol. Bring the final volume to 1 ml with distilled water.
8. Add 50 μl of 1 M Tris–HCl pH 7.5, 10 μl of 1 M EDTA, 876 mg NaCl, 50 μl of 20% SDS and make up the volume to 1 ml.
9. Dissolve 10 mg of proteinase K in 1 ml of TE buffer (10 mM Tris–HCl, 1 mM EDTA).
10. Dissolve 35 g of NaCl (58.44 g/mol) in 80 ml of water and bring up the volume to 100 ml.
11. Dissolve 3.38 g betaine monohydrate (135.163) in 5 ml of distilled water. Filter through a 0.2 μm filter to sterilize and store at 4 °C.
12. For 1 ml of 25 mM dNTP mix add 250 μl of each deoxynucleotide (dATP, dCTP, dGTP, and dTTP), at a concentration of 100 mM.
13. Make a 100 μM stock solution of each primer by resuspension in the appropriate volume of the nuclease-free water. Use the appropriate dilution based on the final volume reaction.
14. Add 250 ml of Tris–HCl (121.14 g/mol), pH 9.0, 714 mg of $MgCl_2$ (95.211 g/mol), 14.5354 g of $(NH_4)_2SO_4$ (132.14 g/mol) and 10 ml of triton x-100 (647 g/mol) and bring the final volume to 500 ml.
15. Dissolve 2.38 mg of $MgCl_2$ (95.211 g/mol) in 1 ml of water.

Acknowledgment

Conflict of Interest: Flora Tassone received funding from Asuragen Inc. and Zynerba for carrying out studies in Fragile X Syndrome. The other author declares no conflict of interest.

References

1. Eichler EE, Richards S, Gibbs RA, Nelson DL (1993) Fine structure of the human FMR1 gene. Hum Mol Genet 2(8):1147–1153
2. Tseng E, Tang HT, AlOlaby RR, Hickey L, Tassone F (2017) Altered expression of the FMR1 splicing variants landscape in premutation carriers. Biochim Biophys Acta Gene Regul Mech 1860(11):1117–1126
3. Maddalena A, Richards CS, McGinniss MJ, Brothman A, Desnick RJ, Grier RE, Hirsch B, Jacky P, McDowell GA, Popovich B, Watson M (2001) Technical standards and guidelines for

fragile X: the first of a series of disease-specific supplements to the Standards and Guidelines for Clinical Genetics Laboratories of the American College of Medical Genetics. Genet Med 3 (3):200
4. Nolin SL, Sah S, Glicksman A, Sherman SL, Allen E, Berry-Kravis E, Tassone F, Yrigollen C, Cronister A, Jodah M, Ersalesi N (2013) Fragile X AGG analysis provides new risk predictions for 45–69 repeat alleles. Am J Med Genet A 161(4):771–778
5. Yrigollen CM, Martorell L, Durbin-Johnson B, Naudo M, Genoves J, Murgia A, Polli R, Zhou L, Barbouth D, Rupchock A, Finucane B (2014) AGG interruptions and maternal age affect FMR1 CGG repeat allele stability during transmission. J Neurodev Disord 6(1):24
6. Tassone F, Iong KP, Tong TH, Lo J, Gane LW, Berry-Kravis E, Nguyen D, Mu LY, Laffin J, Bailey DB, Hagerman RJ (2013) FMR1 CGG allele size and prevalence ascertained through newborn screening in the United States. Genome Med 4(12):100
7. Saldarriaga W, Forero-Forero JV, González-Teshima LY, Fandiño-Losada A, Isaza C, Tovar-Cuevas JR, Silva M, Choudhary NS, Tang HT, Aguilar-Gaxiola S, Hagerman RJ (2018) Genetic cluster of fragile X syndrome in a Colombian district. J Hum Genet 63 (4):509
8. Zlotogora J, Grotto I, Kaliner E, Gamzu R (2015) The Israeli national population program of genetic carrier screening for reproductive purposes. Genet Med 18(2):203
9. Hamlin AA, Sukharev D, Campos L, Mu Y, Tassone F, Hessl D, Nguyen DV, Loesch D, Hagerman RJ (2012) Hypertension in FMR1 premutation males with and without fragile X-associated tremor/ataxia syndrome (FXTAS). Am J Med Genet A 158 (6):1304–1309
10. Summers SM, Cogswell J, Goodrich JE, Mu Y, Nguyen DV, Brass SD, Hagerman RJ (2014) Prevalence of restless legs syndrome and sleep quality in carriers of the fragile X premutation. Clin Genet 86(2):181–184
11. Au J, Akins RS, Berkowitz-Sutherland L, Tang HT, Chen Y, Boyd A, Tassone F, Nguyen DV, Hagerman R (2013) Prevalence and risk of migraine headaches in adult fragile X premutation carriers. Clin Genet 84(6):546–551
12. Hall D, Todorova-Koteva K, Pandya S, Bernard B, Ouyang B, Walsh M, Pounardjian T, Deburghraeve C, Zhou L, Losh M, Leehey M (2016) Neurological and endocrine phenotypes of fragile X carrier women. Clin Genet 89(1):60–67
13. Doherty BR, Scerif G (2017) Genetic syndromes and developmental risk for autism spectrum and attention deficit hyperactivity disorders: insights from fragile X syndrome. Child Dev Perspect 11(3):161–166
14. Hunter JE, Epstein MP, Tinker SW, Abramowitz A, Sherman SL (2012) The FMR1 premutation and attention-deficit hyperactivity disorder (ADHD): evidence for a complex inheritance. Behav Genet 42 (3):415–422
15. Lozano R, Rosero CA, Hagerman RJ (2014) Fragile X spectrum disorders. Intractable Rare Dis Res 3(4):134–146
16. Seritan A, Cogswell J, Grigsby J (2013) Cognitive dysfunction in FMR1 premutation carriers. Curr Psychiatr Rev 9(1):78–84
17. Bourgeois JA, Seritan AL, Casillas EM, Hessl D, Schneider A, Yang Y, Kaur I, Cogswell JB, Nguyen DV, Hagerman RJ (2011) Lifetime prevalence of mood and anxiety disorders in fragile X premutation carriers. J Clin Psychiatry 72(2):175
18. Besterman AD, Wilke SA, Mulligan TE, Allison SC, Hagerman R, Seritan AL, Bourgeois JA (2014) Towards an understanding of neuropsychiatric manifestations in fragile X premutation carriers. Future Neurol 9(2):227–239
19. Roberts JE, Bailey DB, Mankowski J, Ford A, Sideris J, Weisenfeld LA, Heath TM, Golden RN (2009) Mood and anxiety disorders in females with the FMR1 premutation. Am J Med Genet B Neuropsychiatr Genet 150 (1):130–139
20. Jacquemont S, Hagerman RJ, Leehey MA, Hall DA, Levine RA, Brunberg JA, Zhang L, Jardini T, Gane LW, Harris SW, Herman K (2004) Penetrance of the fragile X–associated tremor/ataxia syndrome in a premutation carrier population. JAMA 291(4):460–469
21. Alvarez-Mora MI, Rodriguez-Revenga L, Madrigal I, Guitart-Mampel M, Garrabou G, Milà M (2017) Impaired mitochondrial function and dynamics in the pathogenesis of FXTAS. Mol Neurobiol 54(9):6896–6902
22. Sullivan SD, Welt C, Sherman S (2011) FMR1 and the continuum of primary ovarian insufficiency. Semin Reprod Med 29(04):299–307
23. Cronister A, Schreiner R, Wittenberger M, Amiri K, Harris K, Hagerman RJ (1991) Heterozygous fragile X female: historical, physical, cognitive, and cytogenetic features. Am J Med Genet A 38(2–3):269–274
24. Hagerman RJ, Hagerman P (2016) Fragile X-associated tremor/ataxia syndrome—features, mechanisms and management. Nat Rev Neurol 12(7):403

25. Adams JS, Adams PE, Nguyen D, Brunberg JA, Tassone F, Zhang W, Koldewyn K, Rivera SM, Grigsby J, Zhang L, DeCarli C (2007) Volumetric brain changes in females with fragile X-associated tremor/ataxia syndrome (FXTAS). Neurology 69(9):851–859
26. Brunberg JA, Jacquemont S, Hagerman RJ, Berry-Kravis EM, Grigsby J, Leehey MA, Tassone F, Brown WT, Greco CM, Hagerman PJ (2002) Fragile X premutation carriers: characteristic MR imaging findings of adult male patients with progressive cerebellar and cognitive dysfunction. Am J Neuroradiol 23 (10):1757–1766
27. Grigsby J, Brega AG, Bennett RE, Bourgeois JA, Seritan AL, Goodrich GK, Hagerman RJ (2016) Clinically significant psychiatric symptoms among male carriers of the fragile X premutation, with and without FXTAS, and the mediating influence of executive functioning. Clin Neuropsychol 30(6):944–959
28. Lisik MZ (2017) Health problems in female's carriers of premutation in the FMR1 gene. Psychiatr Pol 51(5):899–907
29. Coffey SM, Cook K, Tartaglia N, Tassone F, Nguyen DV, Pan R, Bronsky HE, Yuhas J, Borodyanskaya M, Grigsby J, Doerflinger M (2008) Expanded clinical phenotype of women with the FMR1 premutation. Am J Med Genet A 146(8):1009–1016
30. Primerano B, Tassone F, Hagerman RJ, Hagerman P, Amaldi F, Bagni C (2002) Reduced FMR1 mRNA translation efficiency in fragile X patients with premutations. RNA 8(12):1482–1488
31. Feng Y, Zhang F, Lokey LK, Chastain JL, Lakkis L, Eberhart D, Warren ST (1995) Translational suppression by trinucleotide repeat expansion at FMR1. Science 268 (5211):731–734
32. Mankodi A, Urbinati CR, Yuan QP, Moxley RT, Sansone V, Krym M, Henderson D, Schalling M, Swanson MS, Thornton CA (2001) Muscleblind localizes to nuclear foci of aberrant RNA in myotonic dystrophy types 1 and 2. Hum Mol Genet 10(19):2165–2170
33. Sellier C, Rau F, Liu Y, Tassone F, Hukema RK, Gattoni R, Schneider A, Richard S, Willemsen R, Elliott DJ, Hagerman PJ (2010) Sam68 sequestration and partial loss of function are associated with splicing alterations in FXTAS patients. EMBO J 29(7):1248–1261
34. Sellier C, Freyermuth F, Tabet R, Tran T, He F, Ruffenach F, Alunni V, Moine H, Thibault C, Page A, Tassone F (2013) Sequestration of DROSHA and DGCR8 by expanded CGG RNA repeats alters microRNA processing in fragile X-associated tremor/ataxia syndrome. Cell Rep 3(3):869–880
35. Todd PK, Oh SY, Krans A, He F, Paulson HL (2013) CGG repeat associated translation drives neurodegeneration in fragile X tremor ataxia Syndrome. Ann Neurol 74:S60
36. Boivin M, Willemsen R, Hukema RK and Sellier C (2018) Potential pathogenic mechanisms underlying Fragile X Tremor Ataxia Syndrome: RAN translation and/or RNA gain-of-function?. European journal of medical genetics, 61(11):674–679.
37. Sellier C, Buijsen RA, He F, Natla S, Jung L, Tropel P, Gaucherot A, Jacobs H, Meziane H, Vincent A, Champy MF (2017) Translation of expanded CGG repeats into FMRpolyG is pathogenic and may contribute to fragile X tremor ataxia syndrome. Neuron 93 (2):331–347
38. Loomis EW, Sanz LA, Chédin F, Hagerman PJ (2014) Transcription-associated R-loop formation across the human FMR1 CGG-repeat region. PLoS Genet 10(4):e1004294
39. Tassone, Flora, and Deborah A. Hall (2016). FXTAS, FXPOI, and Other Premutation Disorders. 2nd ed., Springer.
40. Tassone F, Hall DA (2016) FXTAS, FXPOI and other Premutation disorders. Springer Nature, New York
41. Hall D, Tassone F, Klepitskaya O, Leehey M (2012) Fragile X–associated tremor ataxia syndrome in FMR1 gray zone allele carriers. Mov Disord 27(2):297 301
42. Liu Y, Winarni TI, Zhang L, Tassone F, Hagerman RJ (2013) Fragile X-associated tremor/ataxia syndrome (FXTAS) in grey zone carriers. Clin Genet 84(1):74–77
43. Tassone F, Pan R, Amiri K, Taylor AK, Hagerman PJ (2008) A rapid polymerase chain reaction-based screening method for identification of all expanded alleles of the fragile X (FMR1) gene in newborn and high-risk populations. J Mol Diagn 10(1):43–49
44. Chen L, Hadd A, Sah S, Filipovic-Sadic S, Krosting J, Sekinger E, Pan R, Hagerman PJ, Stenzel TT, Tassone F, Latham GJ (2010) An information-rich CGG repeat primed PCR that detects the full range of fragile X expanded alleles and minimizes the need for southern blot analysis. J Mol Diagn 12(5):589–600
45. Filipovic-Sadic S, Sah S, Chen L, Krosting J, Sekinger E, Zhang W, Hagerman PJ, Stenzel TT, Hadd AG, Latham GJ, Tassone F (2010) A novel FMR1 PCR method for the routine detection of low abundance expanded alleles and full mutations in fragile X syndrome. Clin Chem 56(3):399–408

46. Hantash FM, Goos DG, Tsao D, Quan F, Buller-Burckle A, Peng M, Jarvis M, Sun W, Strom CM (2010) Qualitative assessment of FMR1 (CGG) n triplet repeat status in normal, intermediate, premutation, full mutation, and mosaic carriers in both sexes: implications for fragile X syndrome carrier and newborn screening. Genet Med 12(3):162
47. Strom CM, Huang D, Li Y, Hantash FM, Rooke J, Potts SJ, Sun W (2007) Development of a novel, accurate, automated, rapid, high-throughput technique suitable for population-based carrier screening for Fragile X syndrome. Genet Med 9(4):199
48. Yrigollen CM, Durbin-Johnson B, Gane L, Nelson DL, Hagerman R, Hagerman PJ, Tassone F (2012) AGG interruptions within the maternal FMR1 gene reduce the risk of offspring with fragile X syndrome. Genet Med 14(8):729
49. Bontekoe CJ, Nieuwenhuizen IM, Willemsen R, Oostra BA (1997) FMR1 premutation allele (CGG) 81 is stable in mice. Eur J Hum Genet 5(5):293–298
50. Lavedan C, Grabczyk E, Usdin K, Nussbaum RL (1998) Long uninterrupted CGG repeats within the first exon of the human FMR1 gene are not intrinsically unstable in transgenic mice. Genomics 50(2):229–240
51. Bontekoe CJM, Bakker CE, Nieuwenhuizen IM, van Der Linde H, Lans H, De Lange D, Hirst MC, Oostra BA (2001) Instability of a (CGG) 98 repeat in the Fmr1 promoter. Hum Mol Genet 10(16):1693–1699
52. Peier AM, Nelson DL (2002) Instability of a premutation-sized CGG repeat in FMR1 YAC transgenic mice. Genomics 80(4):423–432
53. Willemsen R, Hoogeveen-Westerveld M, Reis S, Holstege J, Severijnen LAW, Nieuwenhuizen IM, Schrier M, van Unen L, Tassone F, Hoogeveen AT, Hagerman PJ (2003) The FMR1 CGG repeat mouse displays ubiquitin-positive intranuclear neuronal inclusions; implications for the cerebellar tremor/ataxia syndrome. Hum Mol Genet 12(9):949–959
54. Entezam A, Biacsi R, Orrison B, Saha T, Hoffman GE, Grabczyk E, Nussbaum RL, Usdin K (2007) Regional FMRP deficits and large repeat expansions into the full mutation range in a new Fragile X premutation mouse model. Gene 395(1):125–134
55. Brouwer JR, Mientjes EJ, Bakker CE, Nieuwenhuizen IM, Severijnen LA, Van der Linde HC, Nelson DL, Oostra BA, Willemsen R (2007) Elevated Fmr1 mRNA levels and reduced protein expression in a mouse model with an unmethylated Fragile X full mutation. Exp Cell Res 313(2):244–253
56. Berman RF, Willemsen R (2009) Mouse models of fragile X-associated tremor ataxia. J Investig Med 57(8):837–841
57. Alam MP, Datta S, Majumdar S, Mehta AK, Baskaran S, Gulati N, Brahmachari V (2010) Comparative analysis of DNA methylation in transgenic mice with unstable CGG repeats from FMR1 gene. Epigenetics 5(3):241–248
58. Van Dam D, Errijgers V, Kooy RF, Willemsen R, Mientjes E, Oostra BA, De Deyn PP (2005) Cognitive decline, neuromotor and behavioural disturbances in a mouse model for fragile-X-associated tremor/ataxia syndrome (FXTAS). Behav Brain Res 162 (2):233–239
59. Foote M, Arque G, Berman RF, Santos M (2016) Fragile X-associated tremor/ataxia syndrome (FXTAS) motor dysfunction modeled in mice. Cerebellum 15(5):611–622
60. Castro H, Kul E, Buijsen RA, Severijnen LAW, Willemsen R, Hukema RK, Stork O, Santos M (2017) Selective rescue of heightened anxiety but not gait ataxia in a premutation 90CGG mouse model of Fragile X-associated tremor/ataxia syndrome. Hum Mol Genet 26 (11):2133–2145
61. Jin P, Zarnescu DC, Zhang F, Pearson CE, Lucchesi JC, Moses K, Warren ST (2003) RNA-mediated neurodegeneration caused by the fragile X premutation rCGG repeats in Drosophila. Neuron 39(5):739–747
62. Jin P, Duan R, Qurashi A, Qin Y, Tian D, Rosser TC, Liu H, Feng Y, Warren ST (2007) Pur α binds to rCGG repeats and modulates repeat-mediated neurodegeneration in a Drosophila model of fragile X tremor/ataxia syndrome. Neuron 55(4):556–564
63. Iwahashi CK, Yasui DH, An HJ, Greco CM, Tassone F, Nannen K, Babineau B, Lebrilla CB, Hagerman RJ, Hagerman PJ (2005) Protein composition of the intranuclear inclusions of FXTAS. Brain 129(1):256–271
64. Tassone F, Hagerman RJ, Taylor AK, Gane LW, Godfrey TE, Hagerman PJ (2000) Elevated levels of FMR1 mRNA in carrier males: a new mechanism of involvement in the Fragile-X syndrome. Am J Hum Genet 66 (1):6–15

Index

Dalit Ben-Yosef and Yoav Mayshar (eds.), *Fragile-X Syndrome: Methods and Protocols*, Methods in Molecular Biology, vol. 1942, https://doi.org/10.1007/978-1-4939-9080-1, © Springer Science+Business Media, LLC, part of Springer Nature 2019

Printed by Printforce, the Netherlands